Clinical Management of Audiological Disorders: Outcome Measure in Demanding Listening Situation after CI Provision

Clinical Management of Audiological Disorders: Outcome Measure in Demanding Listening Situation after CI Provision

Guest Editors

Matthias Hey
Ulrich Hoppe

MDPI

Basel • Beijing • Wuhan • Barcelona • Belgrade • Novi Sad • Cluj • Manchester

Guest Editors
Matthias Hey
Audiology, ENT Clinic
Universitätsklinikum
Schleswig-Holstein
Kiel
Germany

Ulrich Hoppe
Hals-, Nasen-, Ohrenklinik,
Kopf- und Halschirurgie
Universitätsklinikum Erlangen
Erlangen
Germany

Editorial Office
MDPI AG
Grosspeteranlage 5
4052 Basel, Switzerland

This is a reprint of the Special Issue, published open access by the journal *Journal of Clinical Medicine* (ISSN 2077-0383), freely accessible at: https://www.mdpi.com/journal/jcm/special_issues/VIMW87MIIG.

For citation purposes, cite each article independently as indicated on the article page online and as indicated below:

Lastname, A.A.; Lastname, B.B. Article Title. *Journal Name* **Year**, *Volume Number*, Page Range.

ISBN 978-3-7258-5713-5 (Hbk)
ISBN 978-3-7258-5714-2 (PDF)
https://doi.org/10.3390/books978-3-7258-5714-2

Cover image courtesy of Ulrich Hoppe

Contents

Journal of
Clinical Medicine

MDPI

Editorial

Management of Audiological Disorders in Cochlear Implants: Outcomes in Demanding Listening Situations and Future Perspectives

Matthias Hey [1,*] and Ulrich Hoppe [2]

1 Audiology, ENT Clinic, UKSH Kiel, 24105 Kiel, Germany
2 Department of Audiology, ENT-Clinic, University of Erlangen-Nürnberg, 91054 Erlangen, Germany; ulrich.hoppe@uk-erlangen.de
* Correspondence: hey@audio.uni-kiel.de

1. Introduction

Severe to profound sensorineural hearing loss can nowadays successfully be treated by cochlear implantation. However, cochlear implant (CI) recipients still face communication challenges in several everyday communication situations.

In the early years of provision of deaf patients with a CI, the focus was initially on the perception of suprathreshold speech in quiet [1–3]. Success was defined as better speech understanding along with lip reading. There has been great progress over the last three decades concerning recognition of speech in quiet. Nowadays, the majority of cochlear implant recipients are scoring highly in open-set speech perception in quiet [4,5].

However, although CI recipients are able to perform well in quiet, they are still facing a significant disadvantage when noise is present. In noisy environments, speech understanding of CI recipients deteriorates rapidly as the level of background noise increases [5–7]. With further progress in signal processing in CI systems, suprathreshold speech intelligibility in noise was the next field of great research activities [5–7].

A common measure for the ability of a listener to understand speech in noise is the speech reception threshold (SRT), defined as the signal-to-noise ratio (SNR) where 50% of the speech items are correctly understood. Compared to normal-hearing listeners, the SRT achievable for CI recipients is typically much poorer [8–10].

Modern CI systems try to improve speech comprehension in a noisy situation by utilizing digital signal processing algorithms. A range of sophisticated signal processing algorithms for CI sound processors have been introduced such as conventional beamformer, dynamic range optimization, and spatial post-filter technologies. Each technical approach aimed to improve the speech perception in a specific listening situation like speech in quiet [11,12], speech in noise [13,14], and speech in spatially distributed noise [15–17]. Such noise suppression algorithms are especially successful in stationary noise. For these conditions, an additional significant improvement was found by bilateral/bimodal hearing systems [5,18,19]. The majority of the investigation was performed in stationary noise.

Today, CI systems are not only suitable for hearing and understanding in easy-to-understand dialog situations or in stationary noise. The latter is not representative of typical acoustic listening situations. Patients want to participate in everyday life where noises can be quite different. The 'normal hearing tests' in quiet or in stationary noise characterize everyday listening situations only to a certain extent. In order to describe these demands more precisely, the requirements for ecological validity are summarized as follows: "In hearing science, ecological validity refers to the degree to which research findings reflect real-life hearing-related function, activity, or participation" [20]. The idea of ecological validity is considered as a concept that investigates to what extent the result of a specific audiometric investigation is able to draw a relation to outcomes in hearing situations that can be found in everyday life. One aim of the methodological approach of ecological validity is to reduce the differences between the measurements in the laboratory and the everyday listening environment. This can be achieved by using more realistic acoustic test scenarios [20–22].

Nevertheless, speech comprehension of CI users in contrast to normal hearing listeners decreases when transferring stationary noisy situation to fluctuating noise types [9,10,23]. It must be considered that temporal fluctuations of the interfering noise diminish speech comprehension of the hearing impaired. In particular, patients struggle in the presence of fluctuating babble noise types, commonly found in environments such as schools, restaurants, parties, and shopping centers.

These situations are often associated with greater listening effort, which affects the concentration span for auditory perception and is not assessed by audiometric speech tests [24,25].

According to studies on datalogging in cochlear implant systems, the majority of speech components are in the range below 60 dB_{SPL} [17]. These levels relate to soft speech or speech from a distance. In most studies, the standard target value for understanding monosyllabic words is considered to be 65 or 70 dB_{SPL}. The supplementary comprehension of softer speech below 65 dB has also been the subject of recent studies [26–28].

2. Conclusions

In summary, ongoing research aims to widen the number of CI users who have sufficient speech comprehension in quiet and in stationary noise in general [29]. Further development can be addressed especially in everyday listening situation as follows:

- Enhanced speech comprehension in temporal fluctuating noise, which may also incorporate spatially distributed noise sources;
- Reduced listening effort;
- Audiometric test procedures that better reflect everyday listening situations;
- Improved understanding of soft and distant speech.

Author Contributions: Conceptualization, M.H. and U.H.; writing draft, review and editing, M.H. and U.H. All authors have read and agreed to the published version of the manuscript.

Funding: This research received no external funding.

Conflicts of Interest: The authors declare no conflicts of interest.

References

1. Lehnhardt, E.; Battmer, R.D.; Nakahodo, K.; Laszig, R. Cochlear implants. *HNO* **1986**, *34*, 271–279. [PubMed]
2. Dowell, R.C.; Mecklenburg, D.J.; Clark, G.M. Speech Recognition for 40 Patients Receiving Multichannel Cochlear Implants. *Arch. Otolaryngol.—Head Neck Surg.* **1986**, *112*, 1054–1059. [CrossRef] [PubMed]
3. Burian, K.; Hochmair-Desoyer, I.J.; Eisenwort, B. The Vienna cochlear implant program. *Otolaryngol. Clin. N. Am.* **1986**, *19*, 313–328. [CrossRef]
4. Holden, L.K.; Finley, C.C.; Firszt, J.B.; Holden, T.A.; Brenner, C.; Potts, L.G.; Gotter, B.D.; Vanderhoof, S.S.; Mispagel, K.; Heydebrand, G.; et al. Factors affecting open-set word recognition in adults with cochlear implants. *Ear Hear.* **2013**, *34*, 342–360. [CrossRef]
5. Laszig, R.; Aschendorff, A.; Stecker, M.; Müller-Deile, J.; Maune, S.; Dillier, N.; Weber, B.; Hey, M.; Begall, K.; Lenarz, T.; et al. Benefits of bilateral electrical stimulation with the nucleus cochlear implant in adults: 6-Month postoperative results. *Otol. Neurotol.* **2004**, *25*, 958–968. [CrossRef]

6. Fetterman, B.L.; Domico, E.H. Speech recognition in background noise of cochlear implant patients. *Otolaryngol.—Head Neck Surg.* **2002**, *126*, 257–263. [CrossRef]
7. Müller-Deile, J.; Schmidt, B.J.; Rudert, H. Kieler Erfahrungen mit der Cochlear Implant-Versorgung*. *Laryngo-Rhino-Otologie* **1994**, *73*, 300–310. [CrossRef]
8. Spriet, A.; Van Deun, L.; Eftaxiadis, K.; Laneau, J.; Moonen, M.; Van Dijk, B.; Van Wieringen, A.; Wouters, J. Speech understanding in background noise with the two-microphone adaptive beamformer BEAM™ in the nucleus Freedom™ cochlear implant system. *Ear Hear.* **2007**, *28*, 62–72. [CrossRef]
9. Rader, T.; Fastl, H.; Baumann, U. Speech perception with combined electric-acoustic stimulation and bilateral cochlear implants in a multisource noise field. *Ear Hear.* **2013**, *34*, 324–332. [CrossRef]
10. Hey, M.; Hocke, T.; Böhnke, B.; Mauger, S.J. ForwardFocus with cochlear implant recipients in spatially separated and fluctuating competing signals–introduction of a reference metric. *Int. J. Audiol.* **2019**, *58*, 869–878. [CrossRef]
11. James, C.J.; Blamey, P.J.; Martin, L.; Swanson, B.; Just, Y.; Macfarlane, D. Adaptive Dynamic Range Optimization for Cochlear Implants: A Preliminary Study. *Ear Hear.* **2002**, *23*, 49S–58S. [CrossRef] [PubMed]
12. Holden, L.K.; Brenner, C.; Reeder, R.M.; Firszt, J.B. Postlingual adult performance in noise with HiRes 120 and ClearVoice Low, Medium, and High. *Cochlear Implants Int.* **2013**, *14*, 276–286. [CrossRef] [PubMed]
13. Ye, H.; Deng, G.; Mauger, S.J.; Hersbach, A.A.; Dawson, P.W.; Heasman, J.M. A wavelet-based noise reduction algorithm and its clinical evaluation in cochlear implants. *PLoS ONE* **2013**, *8*, e75662. [CrossRef] [PubMed]
14. Hersbach, A.A.; Arora, K.; Mauger, S.J.; Dawson, P.W. Combining Directional Microphone and Single-Channel Noise Reduction Algorithms: A Clinical Evaluation in Difficult Listening Conditions With Cochlear Implant Users. *Ear Hear.* **2012**, *33*, e13–e23. [CrossRef]
15. Büchner, A.; Schwebs, M.; Lenarz, T. Speech understanding and listening effort in cochlear implant users—Microphone beamformers lead to significant improvements in noisy environments. *Cochlear Implants Int.* **2020**, *21*, 1–8. [CrossRef]
16. Dillier, N.; Lai, W.K. Speech Intelligibility in Various Noise Conditions with the Nucleus® 5 Cp810 Sound Processor. *Audiol. Res.* **2015**, *5*, 69–75. [CrossRef]
17. Dorman, M.F.; Gifford, R.H. Speech understanding in complex listening environments by listeners fit with cochlear implants. *J. Speech Lang. Hear. Res.* **2017**, *60*, 3019–3026. [CrossRef]
18. Henry, F.; Glavin, M.; Jones, E. Noise Reduction in Cochlear Implant Signal Processing: A Review and Recent Developments. *IEEE Rev. Biomed. Eng.* **2023**, *16*, 319–331. [CrossRef]
19. Casarella, A.; Notaro, A.; Laria, C.; Serra, N.; Genovese, E.; Malesci, R.; Auletta, G.; Fetoni, A.R. State-of-the-Art on the Impact of Bimodal Acoustic Stimulation on Speech Perception in Noise in Adults: A Systematic Review. *Audiol. Res.* **2024**, *14*, 914–927. [CrossRef]
20. Keidser, G.; Naylor, G.; Brungart, D.S.; Caduff, A.; Campos, J.; Carlile, S.; Carpenter, M.G.; Grimm, G.; Hohmann, V.; Holube, I.; et al. The Quest for Ecological Validity in Hearing Science: What It Is, Why It Matters, and How to Advance It. *Ear Hear.* **2020**, *41*, 5S–19S. [CrossRef]
21. Steffens, T. Die systematische Auswahl von sprachaudiometrischen Verfahren. *HNO* **2017**, *65*, 219–227. [CrossRef] [PubMed]
22. Blümer, M.; Heeren, J.; Mirkovic, B.; Latzel, M.; Gordon, C.; Crowhen, D.; Meis, M.; Wagener, K.; Schulte, M. The Impact of Hearing Aids on Listening Effort and Listening-Related Fatigue—Investigations in a Virtual Realistic Listening Environment. *Trends Hear.* **2024**, *28*, 23312165241265199. [CrossRef] [PubMed]
23. Zirn, S.; Polterauer, D.; Keller, S.; Hemmert, W. The effect of fluctuating maskers on speech understanding of high-performing cochlear implant users. *Int. J. Audiol.* **2016**, *55*, 295–304. [CrossRef] [PubMed]
24. Meister, H. Speech comprehension and cognitive performance in acoustically difficult situations. *HNO* **2019**, *68*, 171–176. [CrossRef]
25. Pichora-Fuller, M.K.; Kramer, S.E.; Eckert, M.A.; Edwards, B.; Hornsby, B.W.Y.; Humes, L.E.; Lemke, U.; Lunner, T.; Matthen, M.; Mackersie, C.L.; et al. Hearing Impairment and Cognitive Energy: The Framework for Understanding Effortful Listening (FUEL). *Ear Hear.* **2016**, *37*, 5S–27S. [CrossRef]
26. Hey, M.; Böhnke, B.; Mewes, A.; Munder, P.; Mauger, S.J.; Hocke, T. Speech comprehension across multiple CI processor generations: Scene dependent signal processing. *Laryngoscope Investig. Otolaryngol.* **2021**, *6*, 807–815. [CrossRef]
27. Wathour, J.; Govaerts, P.J.; Derue, L.; Vanderbemden, S.; Huaux, H.; Lacroix, E.; Deggouj, N. Prospective Comparison Between Manual and Computer-Assisted (FOX) Cochlear Implant Fitting in Newly Implanted Patients. *Ear Hear.* **2023**, *44*, 494–505. [CrossRef]

28. Dziemba, O.C.; Merz, S.; Hocke, T. Evaluative audiometry after cochlear implant provision. German Version. *HNO* **2023**, *71*, 669–677. [CrossRef]
29. Moberly, A.C.; Bates, C.; Harris, M.S.; Pisoni, D.B. The Enigma of Poor Performance by Adults With Cochlear Implants. *Otol. Neurotol.* **2016**, *37*, 1522–1528. [CrossRef]

Journal of
Clinical Medicine

MDPI

Brief Report

Triple Semi-Circular Canal Occlusion and Cochlear Implantation: A Treatment Option for Single-Sided Menière's Disease with Functional Deafness—A Case Series

Ronny Jacob, Gina Lauer, Arneborg Ernst, Rainer Seidl, Lenneke Kiefer and Philipp Mittmann *

Department of Otolaryngology, Head and Neck Surgery, BG Klinikum Unfallkrankenhaus, 12683 Berlin, Germany
* Correspondence: philipp.mittmann@googlemail.com; Tel.: +49-30-5681-4311; Fax: +49-30-5681-4303

Abstract: The surgical options for patients with single-sided Menière's disease and functional deafness are challenging. Our case series reports the outcomes of surgical treatments of patients with single-sided Menière's disease and functional deafness. These patients have undergone a one-staged occlusion of all semi-circular canals and cochlear implantation. Five patients (four female and one male; 62 ± 8.2 years with a range from 50 to 72 years) with single-sided Menière's disease and functional deafness were included in this study. In all cases, the patients suffered from frequent rotational vertigo episodes for many years. Other treatment options (e.g., medication) had not yet been successful. Preoperatively, the Dizziness Handicap Inventory (DHI) of all patients indicated severe emotional, physical, and functional deficits. Patients showed a functional (near-total) deafness of the affected ear in all cases. All patients were supplied with cochlear implants in combination with a triple occlusion of all semi-circular canals in a one-stage procedure. After a short period of increased dizziness following surgery and after the activation of the cochlear implant and CI rehabilitation (auditory-verbal therapy), vertigo control and an adequate audiological outcome were achieved. The DHI showed a constant decrease after surgery. The combination of a triple semi-circular canal occlusion and cochlear implantation can be an efficient treatment for patients with single-sided Menière's disease.

Keywords: cochlear implant; semi-circular canal occlusion; Menière's disease

1. Introduction

Menière's disease is characterized by recurrent rotational vertigo episodes, tinnitus, and sensorineural hearing loss. The baseline therapy in Europe is oral medication with betahistine or other medication (e.g., calcium antagonists) [1]. In progressive Menière's disease, with conservative treatment, intratympanic gentamicin or intratympanic corticosteroids application can be an option. To achieve both hearing preservation and vertigo control, the best pharmacologic treatment option among the interventions compared may be an IT steroid plus high-dose betahistine, considering that IT gentamicin was found to be associated with benefits toward vertigo control but with potentially detrimental effects on hearing preservation [2,3]. Nevertheless, intratympanic medication cannot always reach an adequate control of the vertigo symptoms [1]. Even more invasive procedures (e.g., endolymphatic sac surgery) cannot safely control the vertiginous episodes in all cases. If those patients additionally suffer from a profound sensorineural hearing loss, the combination of a cochlear implant and a labyrinthectomy or occlusion of the semi-circular canals should be considered [4,5]. Subjects with end-stage Menière's disease, and consequently unilateral hearing loss, suffer from the typical audiological disorders. Decreased sound localization, reduced speech perception abilities, and reduced quality of life due to the loss of binaural hearing can significantly impact the daily routine in patients.

Cochlear implantation (CI) is a worldwide-accepted surgical procedure for an increasing number of patients with severe-to-profound hearing loss. The criteria for cochlear implantation in Germany have expanded over the past decades, nowadays including recipients with unilateral aided residual hearing up to 60% of speech understanding at 65 dB SPL. The plugging of the semi-circular canals can be performed via a transmastoidal approach or via the middle fossa approach for the superior canal. The approach is established and well known from semi-circular dehiscence surgery. Surgery can be performed with only minimal trauma and even without affecting the hearing threshold. Early feasibility studies on hearing preservation after canal plugging were first observed in guinea pigs and later proved in humans. Kontorinis et al. showed that 11 out of 30 patients that were enrolled had significantly improved DHI scores, while hearing did not change significantly. They concluded that the transmastoid plugging of the superior semi-circular canal can safely and significantly improve the vestibular symptoms of patients with SCDS, as well as the auditory symptoms in a substantial number of patients in a hearing-preservation way [6]. The study by the House group showed similar results in a group of 24 ears. Plugging the semi-circular canal is a safe method with vestibular symptom improvement in 35.7% of patients, and word recognition scores did not significantly change postoperatively [7].

Combining vestibular surgery and cochlear implantation is quite a new approach to the neurotological society. Saber et al. performed a single-patient procedure that involved plugging the posterior semi-circular canal and performing cochlear implantation in the ipsilateral ear. The patient had benign paroxysmal positional vertigo with single-sided deafness. The outcome of the procedure was overall successful in terms of vertigo and auditory rehabilitation, but the tinnitus worsened after surgery [8].

While a labyrinthectomy can efficiently control the episodes of vertigo, the procedure also results in complete vestibular deafferentation [9]. In a single-center retrospective study between 2003 and 2019, seventy-two patients underwent unilateral labyrinthectomy. Indication criteria were mostly drop attacks or failure of treatment with intratympanic gentamicin [10]. The mean preoperative word recognition score was 36.4% in the affected ear. The Gruppo Otologico investigated the charts of 22 patients undergoing labyrinthectomy and cochlear implantation in the same ear for intractable vertigo and hearing loss [11]. A total of 67% of the patients had complete resolution of the vestibular symptoms in their operated ear, but speech audiometry after cochlear implantation was not significantly better [11]. They concluded that in Menière's disease with vertigo and severe hearing loss, labyrinthectomy and cochlear implantation can be a reasonable solution, but in the elderly, more failures and postoperative instability are observed.

However, a less destructive approach (canal occlusion) can be particularly helpful for patients who develop Menière's disease in the contralateral ear or for the elderly with an age-related impairment of the balance system. Experimental evidence indicates that a triple semi-circular canal occlusion could be an effective option for controlling episodes of rotational vertigo in Menière's disease [12]. In a small cohort of three patients, Gill et al. performed a triple semi-circular canal occlusion for the treatment of Menière's disease. Two patients showed no effect on hearing whereas one patient suffered a unilateral 30 dB hearing loss. Vertigo control was excellent in two patients. The aim of our study was to investigate vertigo control and hearing performance after a triple semi-circular canal occlusion and simultaneous cochlear implantation in patients with unilateral Menière's disease.

2. Materials and Methods

After unsuccessful conservative treatment to control the episodes of vertigo, one male and four female patients with single-sided Menière's disease [13] underwent surgical treatment. Inclusion criteria were single-sided Menière's Disease, age over 18 years, oral medication for over a year, and severe hearing loss in the affected ear. The mean age was 62 ± 8.2 years with a range from 50 to 72 years. All patients were on medication (from 3 to 19 years) and reported frequent episodes of rotational vertigo as the most impairing symptom (2–3× week on average). The treatment with gentamicin (intratympanic application) or other procedures was declined by the patients. Exclusion criteria included patients younger than 18 years of age, a previous operation in the affected ear, and gentamicin treatment before surgery.

The patients were treated between August 2013 and October 2015 using the identical surgical technique of one-stage cochlear implantation and the occlusion of all three ipsilateral semi-circular canals. For cochlear implantation, a posterior tympanotomy and a round window approach were chosen [14]. Occlusion of the three semi-circular canals was performed before the implantation by reducing the drill speed to 10,000/min. The labyrinth was skeletonized to identify all semi-circular canals. The superior bony layer of the semi-circular canal was drilled down with a diamond burr (2.3 mm) until the endolymphatic duct shone through the last bony layer (blue lining) (Figures 1 and 2). Leaving the endolymphatic duct intact, the temporalis fascia was pushed down in the canal. After sealing with fascia, the canal was filled with bone wax (Figure 3). The area of each canal was covered afterward with a muscle patch and bone pate. Finally, the sealing patch was secured with fibrin glue (Figure 4) [5,15].

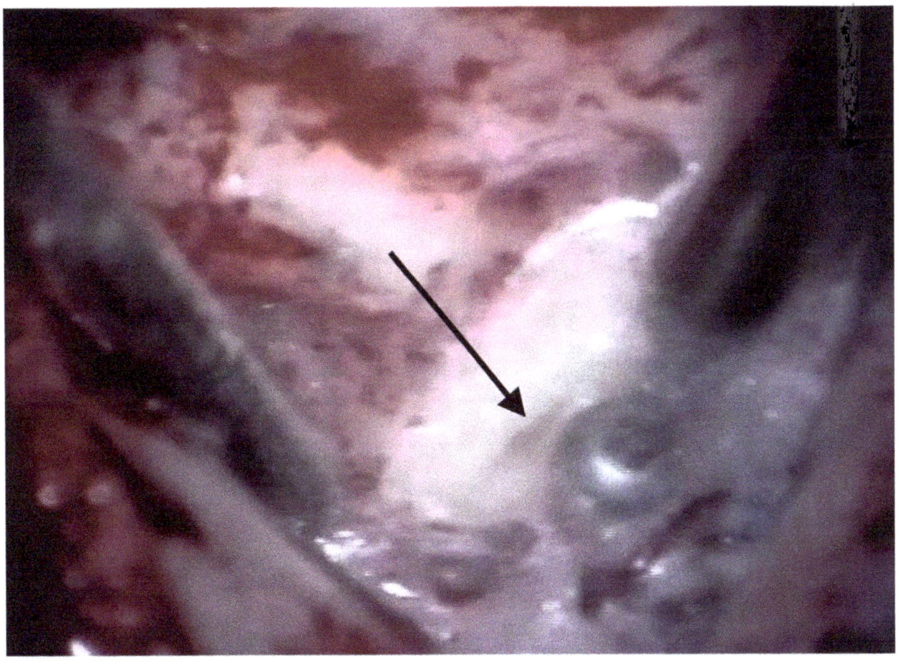

Figure 1. Blue lining of the lateral semi-circular canal with the diamond burr. The arrow points to the lateral semi-circular canal.

The subjective and objective vestibular findings were assessed preoperatively, directly postoperatively, as well as 6–8 weeks and 6 months after surgery. For this purpose, the Dizziness Handicap Inventory (DHI) with its subscales (physical (DHIp), functional (DHIf), and emotional (DHIe)) was used as a reliable and validated instrument for the functional outcome–evaluation [16]. Patients filled in the DHI by themselves. The questionnaire was handed to each patient, who read and filled it by themselves.

Preoperatively, the video head impulse test was performed in two patients (normal responses for all semi-circular canals). Cervical-evoked vestibular myogenic potentials (cVEMPs) were recorded in all patients but could only be elicited in two patients. None of the patients showed spontaneous nystagmus. Caloric tests were not performed.

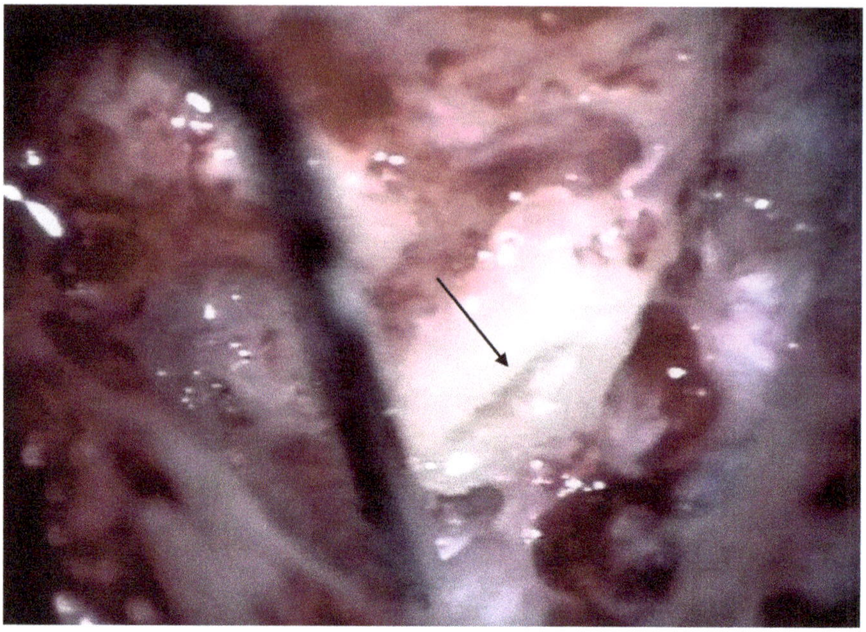

Figure 2. After blue lining of the lateral semi-circular canal, the canal was filled with fascia. The arrow points to the lateral semi-circular canal.

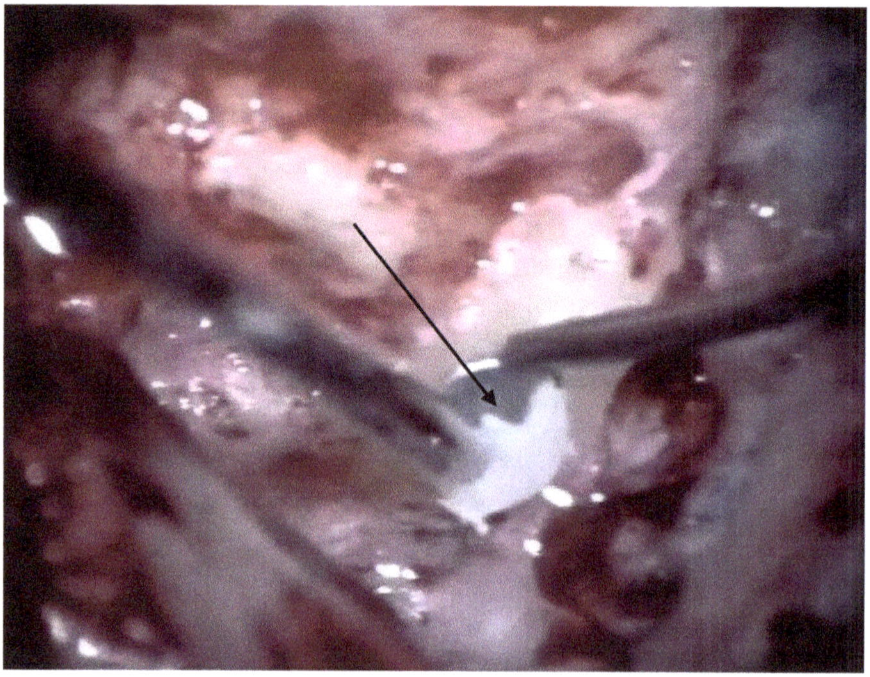

Figure 3. Occlusion with bone wax. The arrow points to the wax applied to the canal.

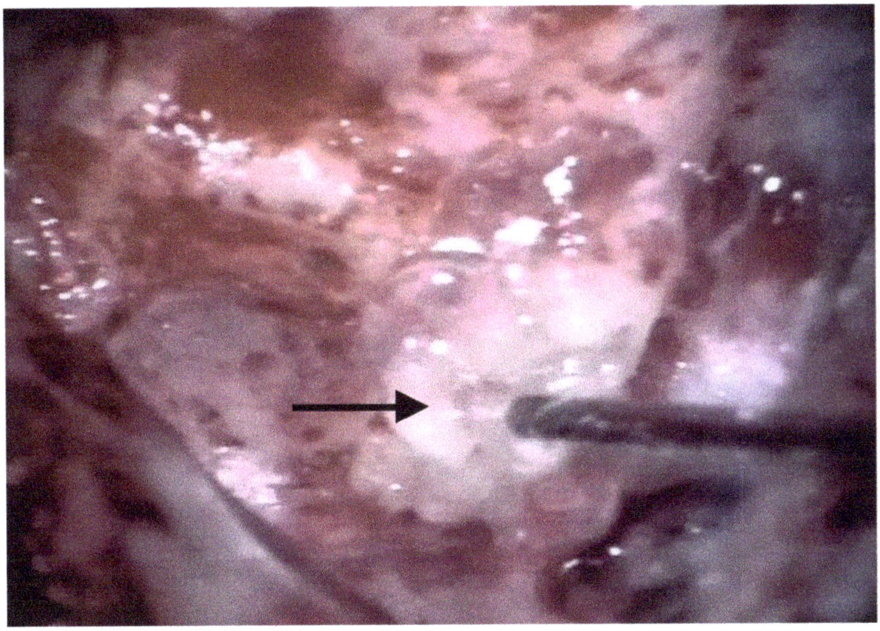

Figure 4. In the last step, fibrin glue was used to seal the plug. The arrow points to the fibrin glue.

The audiological results of the cochlear implantation were assessed by testing numbers and monosyllabic words (Freiburger test) (Table 1). The study was approved by the institutional review board at the BG Klinikum Unfallkrankenhaus Berlin (ukb-hno-2013/4). The study was conducted according to the principles expressed in the Declaration of Helsinki. Statistical evaluation was performed using SPSS (Version 22.0; IBM Co., Armonk, NY, USA). For the comparison between the different DHI scores, a two-way repeated measures ANOVA was run.

Table 1. Patient demographics.

Patient	Age	Sex	Episodes of Vertigo in 1 Year	Mean Pure Tone Average between 500 Hz and 4 kHz	Word Recognition Score	DHI
Patient 1	66	w	24	100 dB	0%	46
Patient 2	50	w	52	95 dB	0%	64
Patient 3	60	m	36	130 dB	0%	46
Patient 4	60	w	20	130 dB	0%	60
Patient 5	72	w	78	130 dB	0%	50

3. Results

Before the surgical treatment was started, the DHI suggested a severe functional, emotional, and physical impairment of all included individuals. Preoperatively, the mean DHI was quantified as serious, regarding the functional (DHIf 20.8 $\pm$ 3.0), and emotional (DHIe 22.4 $\pm$ 6.5) as well as moderate, concerning the physical (DHIp 10 $\pm$ 6.2) deficits (Table 2).

Table 2. Time course of mean DHI score.

Quality	Preop.	Postop.	6 Weeks	6 Months
Physical deficit	10 ± 6.2	8.8 ± 10.7	4.0 ± 4.9	2.8 ± 3.0
Functional deficit	20.8 ± 3.0	16.4 ± 15.9	5.2 ± 5.2	2.4 ± 2.2
Emotional deficit	22.4 ± 6.5	10.8 ± 10.2	5.2 ± 5.8	2.0 ± 3.5

All patients reported a complete cessation of Menière's typical vertigo episodes, but one female patient postoperatively described unstableness instead of the pre-existing vertigo episodes. After revision surgery (labyrinthectomy after three months), she became free of vertigo episodes. The data of this patient included for statistical analysis were those after revision surgery.

Three of the five patients reported an immediate improvement in symptoms (vertigo episodes and unstableness) after surgery. The postoperative DHI of these three patients already indicated a statistically significant decrease in the functional, physical, and emotional subscales during the postoperative hospital stay.

After 6 weeks of compensation, four subjects (and one subject after labyrinthectomy) were almost free of symptoms. Slight vertigo or feelings of insecurity only occurred with challenging activities like sports or hard physical work, as described by some of the patients. Ordinary everyday activities could be performed without any limitations. Six months after the surgery, this status even improved (Figure 5). All subjects did not undergo a specific vestibular rehabilitation program.

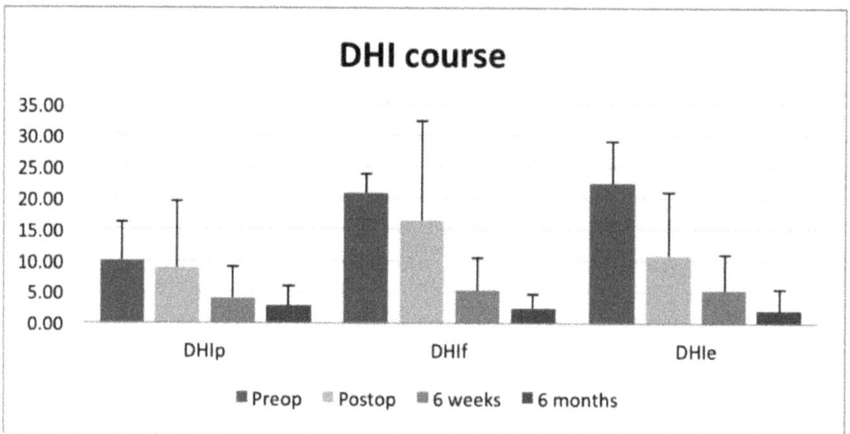

Figure 5. Time course of mean DHI score.

A two-way repeated measures ANOVA was run to monitor the effects over time for DHIp, DHIf, and DHIe. For the DHIp, there was a statistically significant difference in DHIp scores between time points, $F(3, 12) = 25.580$, $p < 0.0005$. Post hoc analysis with a Bonferroni adjustment revealed that DHIp scores were statistically significantly decreased from pre-intervention to six weeks (14.2 (95% CI, 1.238 to 27.162) $p = 0.036$) and from pre-intervention to six months (19.4 (95% CI, 6.511 to 32.289) $p = 0.011$).

For the DHIf scores, there was a statistically significant difference in DHIf scores between time points, $F(1.417, 5.667) = 17.134$, $p = 0.005$. Post hoc analysis with a Bonferroni adjustment revealed that DHIf scores were statistically significantly decreased from pre-intervention to six weeks (10.4 (95% CI, 2.638 to 18.162) $p = 0.017$) and from pre-intervention to six months (18.2 (95% CI, 14.319 to 22.081) $p < 0.005$).

For the DHIe scores, there was a statistically significant difference in DHIe scores between time points, $F(3, 12) = 22.580$, $p < 0.0005$. Post hoc analysis with a Bonferroni adjustment revealed that DHIe scores were statistically significantly decreased from pre-intervention to six weeks (14.2 (95% CI, 1.238 to 27.162) $p = 0.036$) and from pre-intervention to six months (19.4 (95% CI, 6.511 to 32.289) $p = 0.011$).

All patients included in this study had profound sensorineural hearing loss. After cochlear implantation and auditory rehabilitation, all patients reported satisfying speech recognition (Table 3).

Table 3. Individual speech recognition before and after cochlear implantation.

	Preop Monosyl at 65 dB	Postop Numbers at 65 dB	Postop Numbers at 45 dB	Postop Monosyl Words at 65 dB
Patient 1	0	100%	100%	55%
Patient 2	0	100%	70%	75%
Patient 3	0	100%	50%	65%
Patient 4	0	100%	80%	60%
Patient 5	0	100%	60%	25%

4. Discussion

Treatment of vertigo and hearing rehabilitation in patients with Menière's disease is challenging, particularly when the medical treatment options (incl. gentamicin) do not yield sufficient results. In cases of recurrent episodes of vertigo—an ipsilateral profound hearing loss—as well as normal or near-to-normal hearing and proper vestibular function of the contralateral side, ablative inner ear surgery should be considered. Labyrinthectomy is a well-established method for the effective treatment of vertigo episodes or Tumarkin crises caused by Menière's disease with the side effect of cochlear deafness [17]. In a previous study, we reported the combination of labyrinthectomy and simultaneous cochlear implantation in five patients with single-sided Menière's disease and pre-existing ipsilateral deafness [5].

Transmastoid plugging of the semi-circular canals is one surgical option in patients with vestibular symptoms caused by the canal dehiscence syndrome or benign paroxysmal vertigo, as conservative medical treatment is limited. Results from human studies show that vertigo control can be achieved via semi-circular canal plugging, and hearing is not affected [15]. Several studies showed that in 10% to 35% of patients with single-sided Menière's disease, so-called silent contralateral endolymphatic hydrops can be detected [18–21]. Therefore, a labyrinthectomy might severely impair the overall balance and postural control in the long term, so a more selective procedure as described in this paper seems to be more favorable.

Results of unilateral labyrinthectomy vary. The Gruppo Otologico showed that 67% of the patients had complete resolution of vestibular symptoms in their operated ear. On the other hand, speech audiometry after simultaneous cochlear implantation was not significantly better postoperative [11]. They conclude that in Menière's disease with vertigo and severe hearing loss, labyrinthectomy and cochlear implantation can be a reasonable solution, but in the elderly, more failures and postoperative instability are observed [11]. Perkins et al. focus their study on audiological results after simultaneous labyrinthectomy and cochlear implantation in unilateral Menière's disease. Patients with unilateral Menière's Disease who underwent simultaneous labyrinthectomy and cochlear implantation experienced improvements in sound localization, speech understanding, tinnitus severity, and quality of life with the device [22]. In contrast to the study by the Gruppo Otologico, these subjects were younger, but only three subjects were investigated. Our population was slightly younger than in the study by Sykopetrites et al. and more comparable to Perkins et al. Regarding the audiological results, our data seem to underline the data from Perkins et al.

The current data regarding semi-circular canal plugging and simultaneous cochlear implantation are limited. In a small cohort of three patients, Gill et al. performed a triple canal occlusion for the treatment of Menière's disease. Vertigo control was excellent in two-thirds of the patients. Saber et al. showed in a single-patient procedure that the plugging of the posterior semi-circular canal and simultaneously performing cochlear implantation in the ipsilateral ear led to overall success in terms of vertigo control and auditory rehabilitation [8].

Conservative and small invasive procedures such as intratympanic glucocorticoids or gentamicin can be an option in patients with severe vertigo symptoms. Ahmadzai et al. point out that to achieve both hearing preservation and vertigo control, the best pharmacologic treatment option among the interventions compared may be intratympanic steroid plus high-dose betahistine, considering that intratympanic gentamicin was found to be associated with benefits toward vertigo control but with potentially detrimental effects on hearing preservation [2]. Similar results were found by Hao et al. They support the findings, by Ahmadzai et al., that intratympanic gentamicin and glucocorticoids both showed beneficial effects compared with placebo treatment in vertigo management of Menière's disease [2,3]. Lee et al. also found similar results but underline that in their results, a substantial amount of heterogeneity and publication bias was found [23].

Our results underline the hypothesis by Gill et al. and Saber et al. and demonstrate that the functional outcome is similar to a labyrinthectomy with respect to the control of Menière's episodes. The DHI showed a comparable reduction in emotional, functional, and physical impairment. Both techniques led to a highly significant reduction in the DHI to nearly normal values in the long term after a period of at least 6 months of compensation [5]. The functional outcome (DHIf) even followed a better time course in those patients of the labyrinthectomy group [5]. The DHI indicated significantly faster functional improvement after surgery as compared to labyrinthectomy [5]. However, no significant differences in the emotional and physical subscales in the time course were found when comparing both groups. The same holds true for the hearing outcome after cochlear implantation.

The DHI of four out of five patients who underwent triple semi-circular canal occlusion surgery followed a similar time course as the patients who directly underwent a labyrinthectomy. They preoperatively suffered recurrent episodes of vertigo from twice a week up to several times a day. Postoperatively, after a few weeks of vestibular compensation, these patients had a statistically significant reduction in their functional, physical, and especially, emotional subscales of the DHI to nearly normal. Just in one case, no significant improvement of vertigo could be achieved, so revision surgery (labyrinthectomy) had to be performed.

Nevertheless, a triple semi-circular canal occlusion should be chosen as an option before performing a labyrinthectomy for the reasons outlined above. In four out of the five patients in this series, the saccule and utricle (gravity receptors) could be successfully preserved.

Therefore, the least traumatic approach in canal occlusion or revision surgery should be chosen [24–26]. Furthermore, patients gain a benefit from the auditory rehabilitation of the hearing loss with a cochlear implant. Our results, as well as those previously published by Sader et al., strongly advocate for simultaneous cochlear implantation and triple semi-circular canal occlusion in this population due to their substantial benefits. Similar to the mentioned studies, our study is limited to a small number of participants. In addition, the surgeon and the patient are not blinded to the procedure. In all patients, no adverse events were recorded. Neither facial paresis, cerebral-spinal-fluid leak, nor wound infection or infection of the cochlear implant were recorded.

Nevertheless, regardless of the small number of patients, our results demonstrate that simultaneous triple semi-circular plugging and cochlear implantation is a successful and safe procedure in suppressing vertigo symptoms and restoring hearing in unilateral Menière's disease.

5. Conclusions

For patients with single-sided Menière's disease, functional deafness, and frequent episodes of vertigo, simultaneous cochlear implantation with the occlusion of all three semi-circular canals can be an efficient therapeutical procedure. This procedure is as efficient as the labyrinthectomy with simultaneous cochlear implantation in vertigo control. However, the technical aspects of occlusion surgery are more challenging since the preservation of the otolith organs should lead to better postural control postoperatively and would be a huge advantage in those patients who develop a bilateral Menière's disease.

Author Contributions: Conceptualization, R.J. and P.M.; methodology, A.E.; validation, R.J., G.L., L.K., R.S., A.E. and P.M.; formal analysis, R.J. and P.M.; investigation, G.L.; data curation, R.J., G.L., R.S., L.K., A.E. and P.M.; writing—original draft preparation, R.J.; writing—review and editing, R.J., G.L., R.S., A.E., L.K. and P.M.; visualization, R.S. and A.E.; supervision, G.L.; project administration, P.M. All authors have read and agreed to the published version of the manuscript.

Funding: This research received no external funding.

Institutional Review Board Statement: The study was conducted in accordance with the Declaration of Helsinki and approved by the Institutional Review Board ukb/02-2020, 1 March 2020.

Informed Consent Statement: Informed consent was obtained from all subjects involved in the study.

Data Availability Statement: All data are available from the corresponding author.

Conflicts of Interest: The authors declare no conflict of interest.

References

1. Nevoux, J.; Barbara, M.; Dornhoffer, J.; Gibson, W.; Kitahara, T.; Darrouzet, V. International consensus (ICON) on treatment of Meniere's disease. *Eur. Ann. Otorhinolaryngol. Head Neck Dis.* **2018**, *135*, S29–S32. [CrossRef] [PubMed]
2. Ahmadzai, N.; Cheng, W.; Kilty, S.; Esmaeilisaraji, L.; Wolfe, D.; Bonaparte, J.; Schramm, D.; Fitzpatrick, E.; Lin, V.; Skidmore, B.; et al. Pharmacologic and surgical therapies for patients with Meniere's disease: A systematic review and network meta-analysis. *PLoS ONE* **2020**, *15*, e0237523. [CrossRef] [PubMed]
3. Hao, W.; Yu, H.; Li, H. Effects of intratympanic gentamicin and intratympanic glucocorticoids in Meniere's disease: A network meta-analysis. *J. Neurol.* **2022**, *269*, 72–86. [CrossRef]
4. Charpiot, A.; Rohmer, D.; Gentine, A. Lateral semicircular canal plugging in severe Meniere's disease: A clinical prospective study about 28 patients. *Otol. Neurotol.* **2010**, *31*, 237–240. [CrossRef]
5. Doobe, G.; Ernst, A.; Ramalingam, R.; Mittmann, P.; Todt, I. Simultaneous Labyrinthectomy and Cochlear Implantation for Patients with Single-Sided Meniere's Disease and Profound Sensorineural Hearing Loss. *BioMed Res. Int.* **2015**, *2015*, 457318. [CrossRef] [PubMed]
6. Kontorinis, G.; Lenarz, T. Superior semicircular canal dehiscence: A narrative review. *J. Laryngol. Otol.* **2022**, *136*, 284–292. [CrossRef]
7. Goddard, J.C.; Wilkinson, E.P. Outcomes following Semicircular Canal Plugging. *Otolaryngol. Head Neck Surg.* **2014**, *151*, 478–483. [CrossRef]
8. Nami Saber, C.; West, N.; Foghsgaard, S.; Caye-Thomasen, P. Cochlear implantation and simultaneous posterior semicircular canal plugging. *Cochlear Implant. Int.* **2022**, *23*, 358–360. [CrossRef]
9. MacKeith, S.A.; Bottrill, L.D.; Ramsden, J.D. Simultaneous labyrinthectomy with cochlear implantation in patients with bilateral Meniere's disease. *Ann. Otol. Rhinol. Laryngol.* **2014**, *123*, 485–489. [CrossRef]
10. Bergmark, R.W.; Semco, R.S.; Abdul-Aziz, D.; Rauch, S.D. Transmastoid Labyrinthectomy for Meniere's Disease: Experience and Outcomes. *Otol. Neurotol.* **2020**, *41*, 1413–1418. [CrossRef]
11. Sykopetrites, V.; Giannuzzi, A.L.; Lauda, L.; Di Rubbo, V.; Bassi, M.; Sanna, M. Surgical Labyrinthectomy and Cochlear Implantation in Meniere's Disease. *Otol. Neurotol.* **2020**, *41*, 775–781. [CrossRef] [PubMed]
12. Yin, S.; Yu, D.; Li, M.; Wang, J. Triple semicircular canal occlusion in guinea pigs with endolymphatic hydrops. *Otol. Neurotol.* **2006**, *27*, 78–85. [CrossRef] [PubMed]
13. Lopez-Escamez, J.A.; Carey, J.; Chung, W.H.; Goebel, J.A.; Magnusson, M.; Mandala, M.; Newman-Toker, D.E.; Strupp, M.; Suzuki, M.; Trabalzini, F.; et al. Diagnostic criteria for Meniere's disease. *J. Vestib. Res.* **2015**, *25*, 1–7. [CrossRef] [PubMed]
14. Mittmann, P.; Ernst, A.; Todt, I. Intraoperative Electrophysiologic Variations Caused by the Scalar Position of Cochlear Implant Electrodes. *Otol. Neurotol.* **2015**, *36*, 1010–1014. [CrossRef]
15. Wilms, K.; Ernst, A.; Mittmann, P. Hearing Outcomes after Transmastoid Plugging of Superior Canal Dehiscence. *Audiol. Neurootol.* **2018**, *23*, 98–104. [CrossRef]
16. Kurre, A.; Bastiaenen, C.H.; van Gool, C.J.; Gloor-Juzi, T.; de Bruin, E.D.; Straumann, D. Exploratory factor analysis of the Dizziness Handicap Inventory (German version). *BMC Ear Nose Throat Disord.* **2010**, *10*, 3. [CrossRef]
17. McRackan, T.R.; Gifford, R.H.; Kahue, C.N.; Dwyer, R.; Labadie, R.F.; Wanna, G.B.; Haynes, D.S.; Bennett, M.L. Cochlear implantation in Meniere's disease patients. *Otol. Neurotol.* **2014**, *35*, 421–425. [CrossRef]

18. Yazawa, Y.; Kitahara, M. Bilateral endolymphatic hydrops in Meniere's disease: Review of temporal bone autopsies. *Ann. Otol. Rhinol. Laryngol.* **1990**, *99*, 524–528. [CrossRef]
19. Moffat, D.A.; Baguley, D.M.; Harries, M.L.; Atlas, M.; Lynch, C.A. Bilateral electrocochleographic findings in unilateral Meniere's disease. *Otolaryngol. Head Neck Surg.* **1992**, *107*, 370–373. [CrossRef]
20. Conlon, B.J.; Gibson, W.P. Meniere's disease: The incidence of hydrops in the contralateral asymptomatic ear. *Laryngoscope* **1999**, *109*, 1800–1802. [CrossRef]
21. Kitahara, T.; Horii, A.; Imai, T.; Ohta, Y.; Morihana, T.; Inohara, H.; Sakagami, M. Does endolymphatic sac decompression surgery prevent bilateral development of unilateral Meniere disease? *Laryngoscope* **2014**, *124*, 1932–1936. [CrossRef] [PubMed]
22. Perkins, E.; Rooth, M.; Dillon, M.; Brown, K. Simultaneous labyrinthectomy and cochlear implantation in unilateral meniere's disease. *Laryngoscope Investig. Otolaryngol.* **2018**, *3*, 225–230. [CrossRef] [PubMed]
23. Lee, S.Y.; Kim, Y.S.; Jeong, B.; Carandang, M.; Koo, J.W.; Oh, S.H.; Lee, J.H. Intratympanic steroid versus gentamicin for treatment of refractory Meniere's disease: A meta-analysis. *Am. J. Otolaryngol.* **2021**, *42*, 103086. [CrossRef] [PubMed]
24. Borner, U.; Anton, L.; Vibert, D.; Candreia, C.; Caversaccio, M.; Häusler, R. Die Dehiszenz des superioren Bogengangs. In *Proceedings of the Swiss Medical Forum*; J.P. Guyot: Muttenz, Switzerland, 2009.
25. Cheng, Y.S.; Kozin, E.D.; Remenschneider, A.K.; Nakajima, H.H.; Lee, D.J. Characteristics of Wax Occlusion in the Surgical Repair of Superior Canal Dehiscence in Human Temporal Bone Specimens. *Otol. Neurotol.* **2016**, *37*, 83–88. [CrossRef]
26. Kozin, E.D.; Remenschneider, A.K.; Cheng, S.; Nakajima, H.H.; Lee, D.J. Three-Dimensional Printed Prosthesis for Repair of Superior Canal Dehiscence. *Otolaryngol. Head Neck Surg.* **2015**, *153*, 616–619. [CrossRef]

Journal of
Clinical Medicine

MDPI

Article

Tone Decay Reconsidered: Preliminary Results of a Prospective Study in Hearing-Aid Users with Moderate to Severe Hearing Loss

Florian Herrmann Schmidt [1,*], Thomas Hocke [2], Lichun Zhang [1], Wilma Großmann [1] and Robert Mlynski [1]

1 Department of Otorhinolaryngology, Head and Neck Surgery, 'Otto Körner', Rostock University Medical Center, Doberaner Strasse 137-139, 18057 Rostock, Germany; lichun.zhang@med.uni-rostock.de (L.Z.); wilma.grossmann@med.uni-rostock.de (W.G.); robert.mlynski@med.uni-rostock.de (R.M.)

2 Cochlear Deutschland GmbH & Co. KG, Karl-Wiechert-Allee 76, 30625 Hannover, Germany; thocke@cochlear.com

* Correspondence: florian.schmidt@med.uni-rostock.de; Tel.: +49-381-494-8374

Abstract: Among hearing aid (HA) users, there is a considerable variability in word recognition scores (WRSs). This variability is most pronounced among individuals with moderately severe to severe hearing loss. The variability cannot be adequately explained by factors such as pure-tone audiogram, audiogram type or age. This prospective study was designed to investigate the relationship between tone decay (TD) and WRS in a group of HA users with corresponding pure-tone hearing loss. The study population included 22 patients with hearing loss between 50 and 80 dB HL. Aided WRS, unaided WRS and TD were assessed for both ears. TD was found to be frequency-dependent. TD and WRS were correlated, with up to $R = -0.66$. The TD test was revealed to be a feasible method for explaining variability in WRS among HA users with hearing loss below 80 dB. This may contribute to improved differential diagnostics. The TD test may thus offer a better understanding of the limitations of HA use in the context of cochlear implant candidacy assessment for HA users.

Keywords: tone decay; suprathreshold diagnostics; retrocochlear disorders; cochlear implant; hearing aid

1. Introduction

Addressing hearing loss and effectively managing it with hearing aids is vital for improving the quality of life of individuals with hearing impairments. This is especially crucial in cases of severe hearing loss, where the impact on speech comprehension is significantly heightened. A particularly interesting aspect within this field is the variation in speech comprehension among a specific subgroup of individuals characterised by a pure-tone average for thresholds at 0.5, 1, 2 and 4 kHz (4FPTA) ranging from 60 to 80 dB HL, as recent studies have shown [1,2]. It is important to note that this variability in speech comprehension persists even in the presence of adequate hearing aid (HA) intervention. This variability has been found with respect to two measures, namely (i) the 4FPTA and (ii) the difference between the maximum word recognition score, WRS_{max}, and the aided score, WRS_{65}(HA), at a conversational level [1,3–5]. The first concepts to address the discrepancy between WRS and pure-tone thresholds were introduced by Carhart [6]: for word recognition in quiet, this was referred to as "loss of acuity", and a second component caused by impaired processing of audible speech signals was referred to as "loss of clarity". Plomp [7] named these components of hearing loss "attenuation" (class A) and "distortion" (class D). Attenuation can be quantified by pure-tone audiometry. The distortion component characterises the negative impact of reduced temporal and frequency resolution. Furthermore, Plomp [7] stated that the distortion component has a detrimental effect on WRS in quiet as well. Consequently, the distortion component explains the deterioration in speech comprehension that is not expressed by attenuation (4FPTA).

The term "distortion" can be applied to denote individuals who exhibit deficient speech comprehension within the above-mentioned subgroup (persons with 60–80 dB HL 4FPTA). These deficits are thought to have their root causes in disturbed temporal processing and limited frequency resolution of the auditory periphery. A plausible explanatory framework for this phenomenon involves the notion of perceptual decay. In such instances, the perception of loudness diminishes over a brief period, despite consistent sound-level presentation. The tone decay test (TDT), introduced by Carhart [8], entails the presentation of a continuous tone at 5 dB SL (sensation level), with successive increments in intensity until a stable perceptual threshold is achieved. The cumulative increase in intensity resulting from this procedure is termed tone decay (TD).

Abnormal TD may be inferred when attenuation exceeds the threshold of 15 dB. Huss et al. [9] found that abnormal TD becomes more prevalent when hearing loss exceeds 50 dB HL. Importantly, TD is not manifested uniformly across all frequencies and intensities; rather, it is particularly pronounced at higher frequencies compared with lower ones. A decline in loudness perception, known as loudness adaptation, can also occur at higher sound levels, although with less prominence in comparison with stimuli near the perceptual threshold.

The underlying physiological cause of TD has yet to be definitively elucidated. However, the initial observation that low levels and high frequencies are more susceptible to TD led to the formulation of the "restricted pattern" hypothesis [10,11]. This hypothesis suggests that for tones with minimal sensation levels or frequencies that stimulate the basal end of the cochlea, the spatial excitation pattern on the basilar membrane evoked by continuous tones is highly confined. Nonetheless, Wynne et al. [12] posit that TD can be attributed either to direct damage to inner hair cells or to the auditory nerve. Their findings suggest that TD at low frequencies arises from disruptions in ribbon synapses, while high-frequency TD is more likely to be associated with auditory nerve disruptions. Nevertheless, a consensus seems to have formed in that either inner hair cells or retrocochlear structures are involved in the TD phenomenon.

As TD increases, a corresponding decline in both unaided and aided speech recognition can be expected. However, it remains unclear to what extent this decrease can be attributed solely to perceptual decay. Furthermore, it is unclear whether this effect persists even after the provision of an HA and, if so, which frequency range is particularly susceptible to heightened challenges in speech comprehension.

To our knowledge, up to now, there has been no investigation of TD in order to explain the variability in WRS_{max} and WRS_{65}(HA) beyond the impact of 4FPTA. This study was therefore undertaken to investigate a patient cohort characterised by hearing loss (4FPTA) ranging from 50 to 80 dB HL and, after the completion of measurements and discharge of patients, to compare TD with unaided and aided word recognition scores.

2. Materials and Methods

2.1. Patient Characteristics

Twenty-two patients were included in this prospective study: ten males and twelve females. Their mean age was 67.6 ± 14.5 years, ranging from 37 to 88 years. Five subjects had both ears included in this study, resulting in a total of 12 left ears and 15 right ears. The patients visited the clinic for one of two reasons: they were recruited in one of the local hearing aid shops or they visited our clinic for HA evaluation between November 2021 and June 2023. A hearing care professional ensured that the hearing aids were properly fitted for all participants. A technical fitting with an ear mould suitable for the individual's hearing loss was conducted to minimise any impact of processor fitting on performance. The single exclusion criterion was single-sided deafness according to the definition given by Arndt et al. [13].

2.2. Audiological Parameters

All participants underwent audiometric tests in both ears using a clinically calibrated audiometer (AT900, Auritec GmbH, Hamburg, Germany). Pure tones were presented at frequencies of 0.125, 0.25, 0.5, 0.75, 1, 2, 3, 4, 6 and 8 kHz through a headphone (DT48; Beyer, Heilbronn, Germany). To prevent the perception of pure tones through bone conduction in the contralateral ear, masking was initiated when there was a difference of 40 dB between the ipsilateral hearing threshold and the contralateral bone conduction threshold. Subsequently, speech recognition was evaluated by measuring the word recognition score (WRS). In the unaided condition, different sound levels were presented, also through the headphone, to find the highest word recognition score (WRS_{max}). The participant's discomfort threshold served as the upper limit for the levels. A minimum level of 95 dB SPL was presented to all participants. The aided word recognition score, WRS_{65}(HA), was measured in quiet unilaterally at a presentation level of 65 dB sound pressure level (SPL) in free field. The contralateral ear was masked appropriately. The speech test signal (Freiburg Monosyllable Test) was presented frontally in a soundproof room (5 × 6 × 2.5 m).

2.3. Tone Decay Test

For the tone decay test (TDT) [8], an AT900 audiometer was used according to routine procedures, as follows. Before TD testing, an audiogram is obtained. The patient is then familiarised with the TDT measurement procedure: "You will hear a very soft sound. Press the button as soon as the sound is no longer audible" [14].

The TDT is then performed for the frequencies 1, 1.5, 2, 3 and 4 kHz, if possible. This depends on the corresponding threshold with respect to the audiometer limits of 110 dB HL. For the AT900 we used, this procedure is integrated according to the recommendations of Lehnhardt [15]: At each frequency, the starting level is set at 5 dB SL (dB sensation level). The test begins with the presentation of a continuous tone at the starting level for a maximum of 60 s. The patient confirms briefly that this level is audible. When the patient presses the button to indicate that the tone is no longer audible within 60 s, the procedure is repeated. For this, a new starting level increased by 5 dB is presented. The test ends when the patient continues to report audibility for at least 60 s, or when the maximum permissible volume of 110 dB has been reached. The difference between the starting level and the resulting level at the end of this procedure is referenced as TD.

Figure 1 shows an example of measurement in a study participant (right ear) with a very strong tone decay. The left-hand panel (A) shows pure-tone hearing loss (air and bone conduction together with the contralateral masking noise). The right-hand panel (B) shows tone decay, here for 1 kHz, over time. In this example, the last presentation level heard for at least 60 s was 50 dB, and TD at 1 kHz was 25 dB.

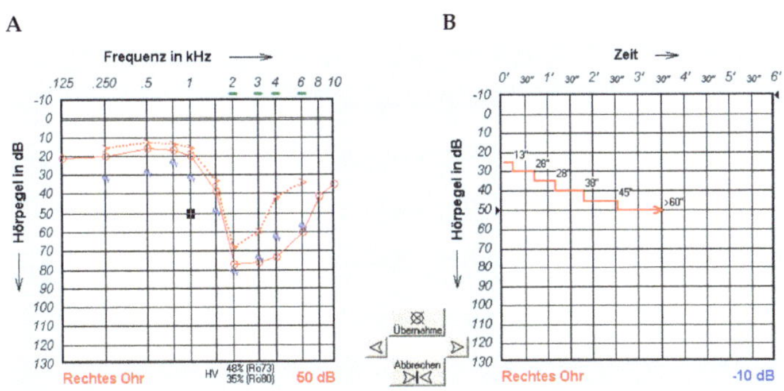

Figure 1. Representative tone decay test performed at 1 kHz and final stimulation at 50 dB HL, 30 dB above hearing threshold. (**A**) Hearing threshold (red circle), the bone conduction threshold (red arrow pointing to the right), and the contralateral masking level (blue wave). (**B**) Change if sound level over time during the tone decay test (TDT).

The performance of the test is limited by the degree of hearing loss due to the 110 dB level limitation and, in the case of asymmetrical hearing loss, by the side difference of the threshold as determined by audiometry conducted before the test (>40 dB was considered excessive). This is because a test involving active masking of the contralateral ear is likely to be less reliable. In addition, with severe hearing loss, auditory fatigue is not always maximally detectable due to the level limitation. This sealing effect must be taken into account when interpreting the results. If tinnitus is present, the test cannot be performed for the frequencies affected.

2.4. Possible Characteristics of Tone Decay Measurements

Figure 2 illustrates a selection of possible characteristics of TD measurements. It underlines the degree to which all the information contained in the TDT is reduced in this first feasibility study, where only the final extent of TD [dB] is evaluated.

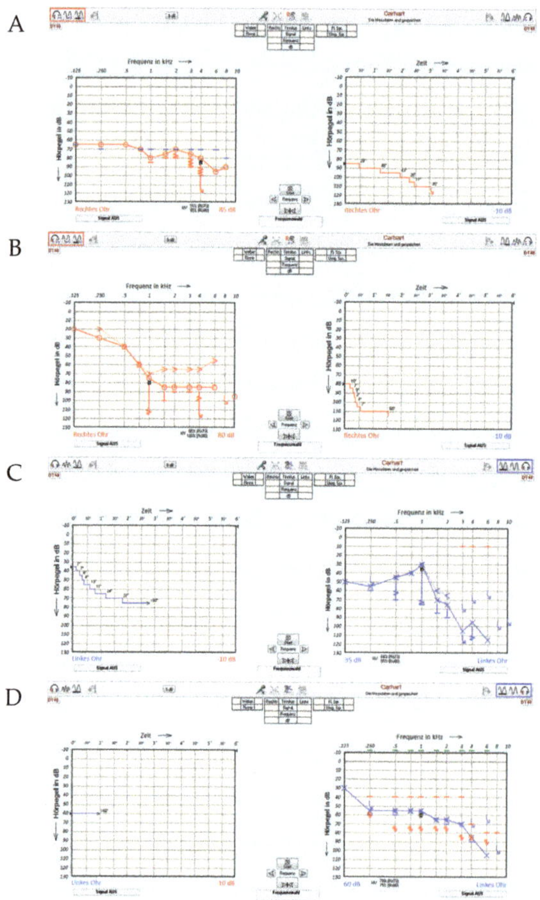

Figure 2. Case examples of different tone decay test (TDT) characteristics. (**A–D**) Case examples. For right-ear cases (red), the graph on the left shows the pure-tone audiogram and that on the right shows the time course of the TDTs. The ordinate corresponds to the presentation level in dB HL. The colours red and blue correspond to measurements of the right and left ear, respectively. The actual test frequency is indicated by a black square symbol on the left while the precise course of TDT is displayed on the right for right ears and vice versa for left ears. The highlighted squares in red and blue in the upper right and left corner visualize the measurement condition.

In case example A, a patient (right ear) with pantonal hearing loss of 4FPTA = 74 dB is presented. TD, here assessed at 4 kHz as indicated by the small black square on the left, is apparently larger than the audiometer limits allowed for measurement. In this case, the TDT yields 25 dB, thereby underestimating the impact of disturbed processing on tone perception. The test time for 4 kHz can be seen in the right-hand part of the figure and was more than 3 min. Case example B shows a patient (right ear) with a steep sloping audiogram and a TD of 30 dB. A special characteristic of this case is the rapid speed of threshold deterioration, as indicated in the right-hand part of Figure 2B. Sometimes, the test tone of 1 kHz was audible more or less for 2 s. Case example C (left ear) shows that this kind of rapid decline is not necessarily connected to a threshold of 75 dB, as in case example B, but may already be apparent at a threshold of 30 dB. As shown in Figure 2C, the test tone was heard for longer with increasing presentation level. However, an audibility of at least 60 s was only reached at 30 dB SL. Finally, case example D shows a patient (left ear) with a moderate sloping audiogram without any TD.

3. Results

The demographic and audiometric data of the study patients are displayed in Table 1.

Table 1. Summary of participants' demographic and audiometric data.

Subjects	Age	Sex	Ear	Ipsilat. 4FPTA [dB HL]	Contralat. 4FPTA [dB HL]	WRS_{max} [%]	WRS_{65}(HA) [%]	Tone Decay at 1, 1.5, 2, 3, 4 kHz [dB]
1	51	f	L	58.8	76.3	0	0	45—n.c.—n.c.—n.c.—n.c.
2	68	m	L	68.8	60.0	55	30	0—n.c.—0—0—n.c.
3	76	m	L	80.0	60.0	90	50	0—10—15—n.c.—n.c.
4	63	m	R	62.5	65.0	65	35	15—n.c.—0—5—10
5	45	m	R	72.5	41.3	75	10	0—0—5—10—30
6	59	m	R	71.3	102.5	0	25	35—10—0—0—25
7	51	f	R	78.8	76.3	45	40	15—n.c.—n.c.—n.c.—n.c.
8	72	f	R	58.8	63.8	75	65	0—5—20—25—20
9	70	f	R	52.5	63.8	90	65	5—5—5—15—15
10	41	m	R	56.3	55.0	65	45	0—n.c.—0—n.c.—5
10	41	m	L	57.5	56.3	85	30	0—n.c.—0—n.c.—0
11	38	f	R	70.0	71.3	80	65	10—0—0—0—10
12	76	f	R	73.8	57.5	15	0	5—15—40—n.c.—20
13	77	m	R	78.8	51.3	75	45	0—0—10—20—10
14	78	f	R	65.0	63.8	65	5	15—n.c.—40—n.c.—45
14	78	f	L	63.8	65.0	45	0	10—n.c.—45—n.c.—55
15	71	f	L	72.5	120	80	75	5—5—5—15—30
16	76	f	R	76.3	63.8	70	0	10—20—25—25—45
16	76	f	L	63.8	76.3	70	15	5—15—30—25—10
17	88	f	R	73.8	38.8	60	35	10—5—5—15—25
18	79	f	R	66.3	62.5	65	10	10—10—20—25—45
18	79	f	L	62.5	66.3	80	25	5—10—20—20—20
19	81	f	R	61.3	57.5	85	60	5—0—0—0—0
19	81	m	L	57.5	61.3	75	45	5—5—5—0—0
20	75	m	L	58.8	52.5	75	70	5—5—5—n.c.—n.c.

Table 1. *Cont.*

Subjects	Age	Sex	Ear	Ipsilat. 4FPTA [dB HL]	Contralat. 4FPTA [dB HL]	WRS_{max} [%]	WRS_{65}(HA) [%]	Tone Decay at 1, 1.5, 2, 3, 4 kHz [dB]
21	57	f	L	72.5	83.8	60	40	0—10—10—0—0
22	78	m	L	63.8	41.3	25	35	0—0—5—20—45

n.c.: not conducted.

The clinical characteristics of the patients did not exhibit any correlation with WRSs. We examined factors such as age, sex, and ear side, comparing them with both WRS_{max} and WRS_{65}(HA). No significant correlation was identified between age and either WRS_{max} or WRS_{65}(HA). Similarly, a two-sided *t*-test for ear and sex characteristics revealed no significant differences.

3.1. Pure-Tone and Speech Audiometry

All ears had moderate to severe hearing loss (Figure 3) and a 4FPTA between 50 and 80 dB HL, with an average 4FPTA of 66.6 ± 7.7 dB HL (mean ± standard deviation). A 4FPTA of at least 30 dB HL was present in the contralateral ear, with an average of 65 ± 17.2 dB HL (Figure 4A). The word recognition score at 65 dB with HA (WRS_{65}(HA)) was 34.1% ± 23.5% (Figure 4B), whereas the maximum word recognition score (WRS_{max}) was 61.9% ± 25.2% (Figure 4C). In almost all cases, WRS_{65}(HA) was below WRS_{max} (Figure 4D).

Figure 3 shows the pure-tone thresholds for the ears included in this study. According to the inclusion criteria, the 4FPTA ranged from 50 to 80 dB.

Figure 4A shows the relationship between the 4FPTAs of the ipsilateral (included case) and contralateral ears. The vast majority of cases show asymmetric 4FPTAs of up to 70 dB. Figure 4B shows WRS_{65}(HA) vs. 4FPTA. The majority (24) of cases exhibit a WRS_{65}(HA) below WRS_{max}. Despite the narrow 4PTFA inclusion band (50 to 80 dB HL), we see a highly variable WRS_{max}, from 0 to 90%, with a variability of the aided scores from 0 to 75% (Figure 4C). Figure 4D shows the relationship between WRS_{65}(HA) and WRS_{max}. For the majority of cases (24/27) WRS_{65}(HA) did not reach WRS_{max}.

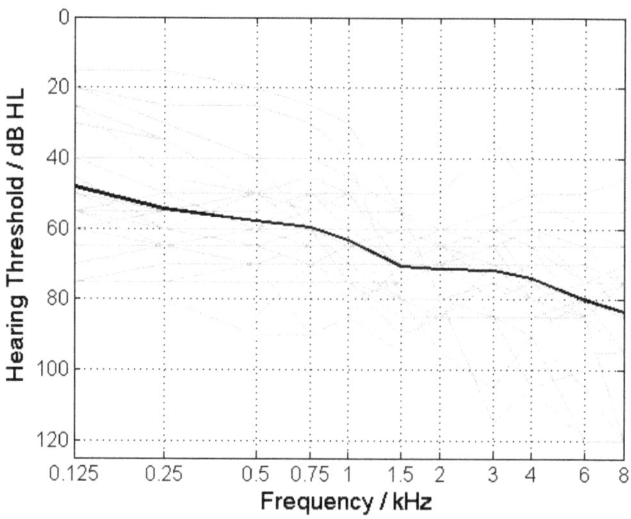

Figure 3. Pure-tone thresholds of the study participants.

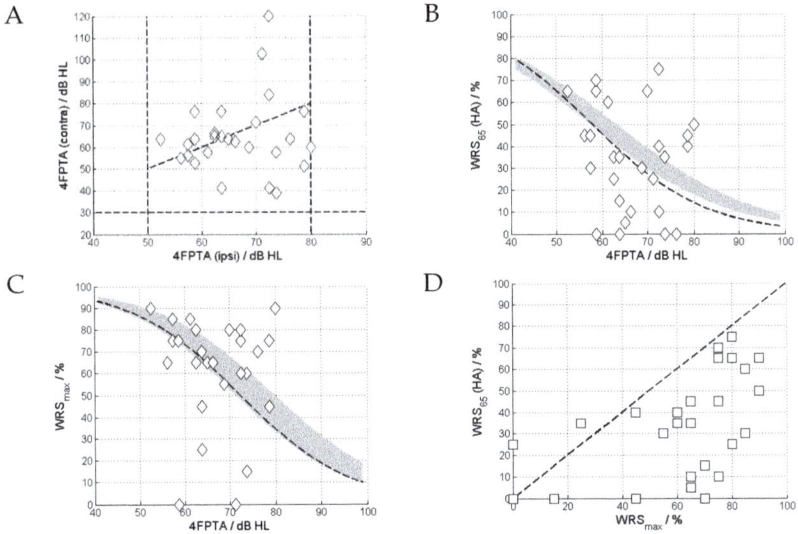

Figure 4. Relationship between four-frequency pure-tone average (4FPTA) and the two word recognition scores. (**A**): Ipsi- and contralateral 4FPTA. (**B**): The aided score, WRS_{65}(HA), plotted against 4FPTA; the grey area shows the average WRS_{max}(HA) as a function of 4FPTA with the corresponding 95% confidence interval [16], and the hatched line shows the logistic regression of the data of this study. (**C**): The maximum word recognition score, WRS_{max}, plotted against 4FPTA; grey area and hatched line as in upper right. The solid line shows the logistic regression of the data of this study. (**D**): Relationship between WRS_{65}(HA) and WRS_{max}.

3.2. Tone Decay

Figure 5 shows the results of TD measurement for the example in Figure 1. The majority of cases showed a TD with higher incidence and amplitude at higher frequencies. The measured TD increased at higher frequencies and resulted in TD_{1kHz} = 8.0 ± 10.6 dB, $TD_{1.5kHz}$ = 6.8 ± 5.8 dB, TD_{2kHz} = 12.4 ± 14.0 dB, TD_{3kHz} = 12.2 ± 10.3 dB and TD_{4kHz} = 21.1 ± 17.2 dB.

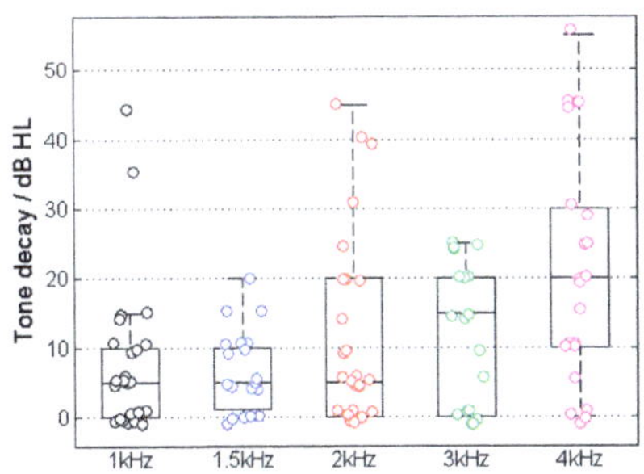

Figure 5. Tone decay at different test frequencies.

The correlations between the TDs for each frequency and speech recognition for both WRS_{65}(HA) and WRS_{max} were investigated. Significant correlations were found for WRS_{65}(HA) and $TD_{1.5kHz}$ ($R = -0.60$, $p < 0.01$) and TD_{2kHz} ($R = -0.63$, $p < 0.001$) (Figure 6) as well as WRS_{max} and TD_{1kHz} ($R = -0.66$, $p < 0.001$). The same result was obtained from the frequency-specific comparison after the subjects had been grouped into normal and abnormal TD, resulting in WRS_{65}(HA) and $TD_{1.5kHz}$ ($p = 0.005$) and TD_{2kHz} ($p = 0.006$) as well as WRS_{max} and TD_{1kHz} ($p = 0.006$).

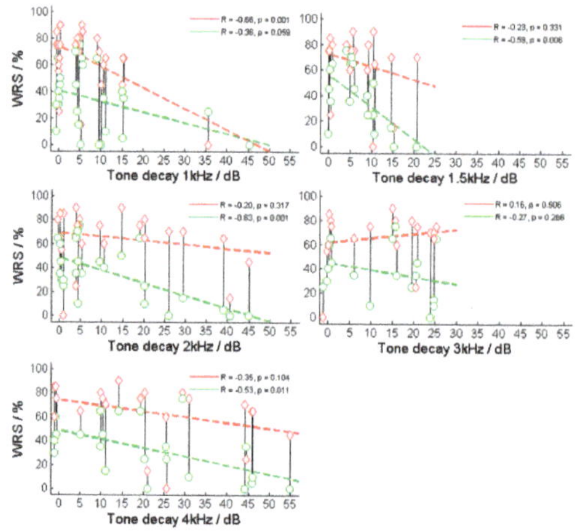

Figure 6. Relation between maximum and aided word recognition scores (WRS_{max} and WRS_{65}(HA)) and tone decay (TD) at different frequencies. The red diamonds and lines correspond to the relationship between TD and WRS_{max}, while the green circles and lines correspond to the relationship between TD and WRS_{65}(HA).

Figure 5 shows the relationship between the two WRSs (WRS_{max} and WRS_{65}(HA)) and TD for various test frequencies.

4. Discussion

4.1. Tone Decay and Speech Comprehension

In this study, we explored the relationship between speech comprehension in individuals with moderately severe to severe hearing loss (4FPTA = 50–80 dB HL) and tone decay within the frequency range 1–4 kHz. Our hypothesis posits that a portion of the considerable variability in speech comprehension within this threshold range for hearing loss could be elucidated by factors such as tone decay (TD). The large variability (90 percentage points for WRS_{max} and 75 percentage points for WRS_{65}(HA)) in the inclusion range for this study (50–80 dB HL) corresponds to previously reported WRSs in a larger population of HA users [1,3–5,17,18]. This applies also to the difference between maximum and aided WRSs. We conclude that the results of our study are applicable to the population of hearing aid users typical for an ENT department of a maximum-care hospital with a cochlear implant programme.

The key finding of this study is the negative correlation between TD and speech comprehension. A consistent trend is evident across all frequencies, with the 1–2 kHz range demonstrating the most clearly significant correlation. This finding aligns with expectations, considering the critical importance of this frequency range for speech comprehension. Moreover, our investigation may indicate that the impact of TD on speech comprehension is more pronounced when using HAs compared with situations without them in the frequency range between 1.5 and 3 kHz. Notably, during the unaided speech comprehension test, we examined WRS_{max} at levels typically reaching the discomfort level, whereas in the aided test, speech was assessed at 65 dB SPL in free field. In cases with unstable thresholds, which correspond to higher tone decays, the fitting of the HA to the threshold becomes imprecise, resulting in inaccurate assumptions for frequency-specific amplification in the presence of TD. Additionally, TD occurs more rapidly with active HAs, as they consistently stimulate close to and beyond the threshold. In contrast, WRS_{max} appears more resilient against TD, possibly owing to the consideration of several levels within the measurement paradigm.

This outcome highlights the constraints of traditional approaches to HA programming when confronted with TD, shedding light on why this particular patient group may no longer be deemed suitable for HA fitting and might be more inclined toward consideration for cochlear implant (CI) fitting. Nevertheless, exploring alternative fitting strategies that take TD into account is a plausible avenue. Such strategies would require the recalibration of thresholds and corresponding amplification, tailored to the frequency-specific challenges posed by TD. To achieve this, the frequency- and level-specific temporal trajectory of TD would need to be recorded individually, coupled with an understanding of possible threshold recovery processes.

4.2. Application of Tone Decay Assessment in a Changing Patient Population

One important aspect of HA evaluation in our clinic is the assessment of cochlear implant (CI) candidacy. The most recent German CI guidelines [19] support CI implantation up to $WRS_{65}(HA) \leq 60\%$ regardless of pure-tone thresholds. In the past decade, this has led to a growing number of CI candidates among cases with considerable aided WRS [20–23]. Together with a higher preoperative $WRS_{65}(HA)$, this also extends CI provisions to some patients with a 4FPTA of 50 dB HL [20–23]. These patient characteristics would allow for improved preoperative differential diagnoses in CI candidates with good 4FPTA and poor WRS. Since some of these diagnostic tests for CIs (of which TDT is one example) require a sufficient amount of residual hearing, TDT may offer a chance—and may meet the clinical need—to explain the variability in $WRS_{65}(HA)$. If, for instance, a CI candidate shows a PTA and disproportional loss in aided speech recognition, a TDT should be applied. A considerable TD may limit the residual dynamic of the patient's HA or alternative hearing system to such a degree that a CI can be considered a better alternative [16,24–26]. Potentially, the decision to conduct another HA trial can be based on such differential diagnostics.

Additionally, the nature of poor performance in a CI-fitted population is not yet understood [27]. For example, recent studies [28–30] have devoted considerable effort to showing that various factors—including genetic disposition, aetiology, and comorbidities—have an effect on CI outcome. Furthermore, preoperative audiometric assessment in clinical routine [19] potentially provides prognostic value [20–23]. However, we still see an urgent need for further improvement in preoperative audiometric assessments. Supra-threshold diagnostic tests, such as TDT and other measurements, as earlier applied for topodiagnostics [31,32] in the presence of less sophisticated imaging resources, could experience a renaissance in the preoperative assessment of CI candidates. Retrocochlear lesions can be ruled out by modern imaging, which is superior to audiometry for this purpose [33]. Other retrocochlear deficits can be quantified by the reapplication of established supra-threshold tests and available objective measures [27,34,35]. In the long term, it might be possible to determine a correlation between these additional preoperative diagnostic results and speech recognition with a CI. A clustering according to different patient characteristics may help to solve the enigma of poor performance [27]. If preoperative TD also partially explains the variability in word recognition with CI, then it should be included in future studies. In the past, TDTs were already performed in CI recipients [36,37]. Wable et al. [36] concluded that TD might facilitate further study of the condition of the auditory system in CI recipients as well as help to follow up on possible retrocochlear damage and to link TD to neural survival. Wasman et al. [37] highlighted the potential use of TDTs to explain the spread of outcomes in CI recipients but, because of the small number of study participants, they did not draw clear conclusions. It appears that, together with TD in CI recipients, the preoperative assessment of TD can contribute to a better understanding of the above relationships.

4.3. Limits of this Study and Feasibility

The assessment of TD was essentially feasible in our study population. However, the TD assessment took up to 1.5 h. The procedure was perceived as demanding by some of the more elderly study participants. In our experience, some patients may require a more extensive introduction to the test procedure as well as a training run. Furthermore, before the TDT, a precise determination of audiometric thresholds is required; this too can be a challenging task for some patients. Some recipients had difficulties in listening to pure-tone presentations for longer periods. Additionally, tinnitus can be expected to have a detrimental influence on the precision of TDTs. For some patients, the perception of the (pure) test tone may change into a noise-like perception, which can be considered a symptom of possible neural pathologies [14]. Finally, in some patients, two ceiling effects potentially limit the diagnostic value. The first refers to the ceiling of the speech test, while the second may occur in cases where 4FPTA is already poor and the full impact of TD cannot be assessed owing to audiometer limits or the fact that an uncomfortable presentation level has already been reached. To follow up on the results reported here, we plan to continue this study. An increased number of study participants would allow for analysis with respect to even more different patient characteristics, as indicated by the measurement examples in Figure 2.

5. Conclusions

The tone decay test is a feasible method for determining tone decay and may contribute to explaining the variability of word recognition scores in hearing aid users with hearing loss in the range 50–80 dB. In cases of disproportionally low aided scores, the tone decay test represents a valuable complement for differential diagnostics. It may provide a better understanding of the limits of hearing aid use in patients considered for cochlear implantation.

Author Contributions: Conceptualisation, F.H.S., W.G. and R.M.; methodology, F.H.S.; software, F.H.S.; validation and formal analysis, F.H.S.; investigation, F.H.S.; resources, F.H.S.; data curation, F.H.S.; writing—original draft preparation, F.H.S. and T.H.; writing—review and editing, F.H.S., T.H., L.Z., W.G. and R.M.; visualisation, F.H.S.; supervision, R.M.; project administration, R.M., W.G. and F.H.S.; funding acquisition, R.M. and F.H.S. All authors have read and agreed to the published version of the manuscript.

Funding: This research was partially funded by Cochlear™ Research and Development Limited, Addlestone UK, grant number IIR-2347.

Institutional Review Board Statement: Ethical approval by the Ethics Committee at Rostock University Medical Center. Approval code: A 2021-0223. Approval date: 18 October 2021. This study was registered in the German Clinical Trials Register under DRKS00032357, https://www.drks.de/DRKS00032357 (last updated on 24 November 2023).

Informed Consent Statement: Informed consent was obtained from all subjects involved in the study.

Data Availability Statement: Supporting raw data may be obtained through special request from the corresponding autor.

Conflicts of Interest: F.H.S., R.M. and W.G. received funding for other projects supported by different medical device companies. T.H. is an employee of Cochlear Deutschland GmbH & Co. The other authors declare no conflict of interest.

References

1. Dörfler, C.; Hocke, T.; Hast, A.; Hoppe, U. Speech recognition with hearing aids for 10 standard audiograms: English version. *HNO* **2020**, *68*, 93–99. [CrossRef]
2. Engler, M.; Digeser, F.; Hoppe, U. Effectiveness of hearing aid provision for severe hearing loss. *HNO* **2022**, *70*, 520–532. [CrossRef] [PubMed]
3. McRackan, T.R.; Ahlstrom, J.B.; Clinkscales, W.B.; Meyer, T.A.; Dubno, J.R. Clinical Implications of Word Recognition Differences in Earphone and Aided Conditions. *Otol. Neurotol.* **2016**, *37*, 1475–1481. [CrossRef]
4. McRackan, T.R.; Fabie, J.E.; Burton, J.A.; Munawar, S.; Holcomb, M.A.; Dubno, J.R. Earphone and Aided Word Recognition Differences in Cochlear Implant Candidates. *Otol. Neurotol.* **2018**, *39*, e543–e549. [CrossRef] [PubMed]
5. Franks, Z.G.; Jacob, A. The speech perception gap in cochlear implant patients. *Cochlear Implant. Int.* **2019**, *20*, 176–181. [CrossRef] [PubMed]
6. Carhart, R. Basic principles of speech audiometry. *Acta Otolaryngol.* **1951**, *40*, 62–71. [CrossRef]
7. Plomp, R. Auditory handicap of hearing impairment and the limited benefit of hearing aids. *J. Acoust. Soc. Am.* **1978**, *63*, 533–549. [CrossRef]

8. Carhart, R. Clinical determination of abnormal auditory adaptation. *AMA Arch. Otolaryngol.* **1957**, *65*, 32–39. [CrossRef]
9. Huss, M.; Moore, B.C. Tone decay for hearing-impaired listeners with and without dead regions in the cochlea. *J. Acoust. Soc. Am.* **2003**, *114*, 3283–3294. [CrossRef]
10. Scharf, B. Loudness adaptation. In *Hearing Research and Theory*; Tobias, J.V., Schubert, E.D., Eds.; Academic Press: New York, NY, USA, 1983; Volume 2, pp. 1–56.
11. Miśkiewicz, A.; Scharf, B.; Hellman, R.; Meiselman, C. Loudness adaptation at high frequencies. *J. Acoust. Soc. Am.* **1993**, *94*, 1281–1286. [CrossRef]
12. Wynne, D.P.; Zeng, F.G.; Bhatt, S.; Michalewski, H.J.; Dimitrijevic, A.; Starr, A. Loudness adaptation accompanying ribbon synapse and auditory nerve disorders. *Brain* **2013**, *136*, 1626–1638. [CrossRef] [PubMed]
13. Arndt, S.; Laszig, R.; Aschendorff, A.; Hassepass, F.; Beck, R.; Wesarg, T. Cochlear implant treatment of patients with single-sided deafness or asymmetric hearing loss. *HNO* **2017**, *65*, 98–108. [CrossRef] [PubMed]
14. Mrowinski, D.; Scholz, G. *Audiometrie Eine Anleitung Für Die Praktische Hörprüfung*, 5th ed.; Georg Thieme Verlag: Stuttgart, Germany, 2017; p. 58ff. ISBN 978-3-13-240107-5.
15. Lehnhardt, E. Adaptation und Hörermüdung. In *Praxis der Audiometrie*, 8th ed.; Lehnhardt, E., Laszig, R., Eds.; Thieme: Stuttgart, Germany, 2001; p. 153ff.
16. Hoppe, U.; Hast, A.; Hocke, T. Audiometry-Based Screening Procedure for Cochlear Implant Candidacy. *Otol. Neurotol.* **2015**, *36*, 1001–1005. [CrossRef] [PubMed]
17. Kronlachner, M.; Baumann, U.; Stover, T.; Weissgerber, T. Investigation of the quality of hearing aid provision in seniors considering cognitive functions. *Laryngorhinootologie* **2018**, *97*, 852–859. [CrossRef]
18. Beyer, A.; Rieck, J.H.; Mewes, A.; Dambon, J.A.; Hey, M. Extended preoperative speech audiometric diagnostics for cochlear implant treatment. *HNO* **2023**, *71*, 779–786. [CrossRef] [PubMed]
19. AWMF. Leitlinien: Cochlea-Implantat Versorgung und Zentral-Auditorische Implantate. 2020. Available online: https://www.awmf.org/uploads/tx_szleitlinien/017-071l_S2k_Cochlea-Implantat-Versorgung-zentral-auditorische-Implantate_2020-12.pdf (accessed on 1 June 2023).
20. Hoppe, U.; Hocke, T.; Hast, A.; Iro, H. Cochlear Implantation in Candidates With Moderate-to-Severe Hearing Loss and Poor Speech Perception. *Laryngoscope* **2021**, *131*, E940–E945. [CrossRef]
21. Thangavelu, K.; Nitzge, M.; Weiß, R.M.; Mueller-Mazzotta, J.; Stuck, B.A.; Reimann, K. Role of cochlear reserve in adults with cochlear implants following post-lingual hearing loss. *Eur. Arch. Otorhinolaryngol.* **2022**, *280*, 1063–1071. [CrossRef]
22. Rieck, J.H.; Beyer, A.; Mewes, A.; Caliebe, A.; Hey, M. Extended Preoperative Audiometry for Outcome Prediction and Risk Analysis in Patients Receiving Cochlear Implants. *J. Clin. Med.* **2023**, *12*, 3262. [CrossRef] [PubMed]
23. Hoppe, U.; Hast, A.; Hocke, T. Validation of a predictive model for speech discrimination after cochlear implant provision. *HNO* **2023**, *71*, 53–59. [CrossRef]
24. Zwartenkot, J.W.; Snik, A.D.F.M.; Mylanus, E.A.; Mulder, J.J. Amplification options for patients with mixed hearing loss. *Otol. Neurotol.* **2014**, *35*, 221–226. [CrossRef]
25. Rahne, T.; Plontke, S.K. Device-based treatment of mixed hearing loss: An audiological comparison of current hearing systems. *HNO* **2016**, *64*, 91–100. [CrossRef] [PubMed]
26. Rahne, T. Physical audiological principles of implantable hearing systems: About power transmission, coupling and power output. *HNO* **2021**, *69*, 475–482. [CrossRef] [PubMed]
27. Moberly, A.C.; Bates, C.; Harris, M.S.; Pisoni, D.B. The Enigma of Poor Performance by Adults with Cochlear Implants. *Otol. Neurotol.* **2016**, *37*, 1522–1528. [CrossRef] [PubMed]
28. Goudey, B.; Plant, K.; Kiral, I.; Jimeno-Yepes, A.; Swan, A.; Gambhir, M.; Büchner, A.; Kludt, E.; Eikelboom, R.H.; Sucher, C.; et al. A MultiCenter Analysis of Factors Associated with Hearing Outcome for 2,735 Adults with Cochlear Implants. *Trends Hear.* **2021**, *25*, 23312165211037525. [CrossRef] [PubMed]
29. Lee, E.; Pisa, J.; Hochman, J. Comorbidity associated with worse outcomes in a population of limited cochlear implant performers. *Laryngoscope Investig. Otolaryngol.* **2023**, *8*, 230–235. [CrossRef] [PubMed]
30. Tropitzsch, A.; Schade-Mann, T.; Gamerdinger, P.; Dofek, S.; Schulte, B.; Schulze, M.; Fehr, S.; Biskup, S.; Haack, T.B.; Stöbe, P.; et al. Variability in Cochlear Implantation Outcomes in a Large German Cohort with a Genetic Etiology of Hearing Loss. *Ear Hear.* **2023**, *44*, 1464–1484. [CrossRef] [PubMed]
31. Thomsen, J.; Terkildsen, K. Audiological findings in 125 cases of acoustic neuromas. *Acta Otolaryngol.* **1975**, *80*, 353–361. [CrossRef]
32. Gertner, A.B. Site of lesion testing findings in a routine test battery. *Am. J. Otol.* **1981**, *2*, 219–222.
33. Strasilla, C.; Synchra, V. Imaging-based diagnosis of vestibular schwannoma. *HNO* **2017**, *65*, 373–380. [CrossRef]
34. Hoth, S.; Dziemba, O.C. The Role of Auditory Evoked Potentials in the Context of Cochlear Implant Provision. *Otol. Neurotol.* **2017**, *38*, e522–e530. [CrossRef]
35. Dziemba, O.C.; Hocke, T.; Müller, A. EABR on cochlear implant—Measurements from clinical routine compared to reference values. *GMS Z Audiol* **2022**, *4*, Doc05. [CrossRef]

36. Wable, J.; Frachet, B.; Gallego, S. Tone decay at threshold with auditory electrical stimulation in digisonic cochlear implantees. *Audiology* **2001**, *40*, 265–271. [CrossRef] [PubMed]
37. Wasmann, J.A.; van Eijl, R.H.M.; Versnel, H.; van Zanten, G.A. Assessing auditory nerve condition by tone decay in deaf subjects with a cochlear implant. *Int. J. Audiol.* **2018**, *57*, 864–871. [CrossRef] [PubMed]

Journal of
Clinical Medicine

MDPI

Article

The Effects of Stimulus Repetition Rate on Electrically Evoked Auditory Brainstem Potentials in Postlingually Deafened Adult Cochlear Implant Recipients

Oliver C. Dziemba [1,*], Tina Brzoska [1], Thomas Hocke [2] and Friedrich Ihler [1]

1 Departement of Otorhinolarygology, Head and Neck Surgery, University Medicine Greifswald, 17475 Greifswald, Germany; tina.brzoska@med.uni-greifswald.de (T.B.); friedrich.ihler@med.uni-greifswald.de (F.I.)
2 Cochlear Deutschland GmbH & Co. KG, 30539 Hannover, Germany; thocke@cochlear.com
* Correspondence: oliver.dziemba@med.uni-greifswald.de; Tel.: +49-3834-86-6289

Abstract: Background: By using outcome prediction scores, it is possible to distinguish between good and poor performers with cochlear implants (CI) after CI implantation. The reasons for poor performance, despite good basic conditions, can be manifold. On the one hand, the postoperative fitting may be inadequate; on the other, neurophysiological disease processes may impair speech understanding with a CI. These disease processes are not yet fully understood. In acoustics, it is known that the auditory brainstem responses (ABR) and their latencies and amplitudes allow differential diagnosis based on reference values for normal-hearing individuals. The aim of this study was to provide reference values for electrically evoked brainstem responses (EABRs) in terms of rate-dependent latencies and amplitudes. **Methods:** 20 ears of 18 experienced adult CI recipients with a predicted and measured good postoperative word recognition score were recruited from the clinic's patient pool. In the same stimulation mode and intensity we measured latencies and interpeak-latencies of EABRs and electrically evoked compound action potentials (ECAPs). With a defined supra-threshold stimulation intensity above the individual ECAP threshold, we applied stimulation at several rates between 11 and 91 stimuli per second. **Results:** We found rate dependences for EABR latency t3 and t5 in the order of 0.19 ms and 0.37 ms, respectively, while ECAP was not affected by rate. Correspondingly, the interpeak intervals' rate dependences for t5 − t1, t5 − t3 and t3 − t1 were of the order of 0.37 ms, 0.18 ms and 0.19 ms. Comparing the EABR amplitudes between the stimulation rates 11/s and 81/s, we found that at 81/s the amplitudes were significantly reduced down: to 73% for A3 and 81% for A5. These rate dependences of latency and amplitude in EABR have characteristics comparable to those of acoustic ABR. **Conclusions:** These data may serve to provide reference values for EABR and ECAP latencies, interpeak intervals and amplitudes with respect to stimulation rate. Altered response patterns of ECAPs and EABRs to normalised stimulation modes could be used in the future to describe and classify neuropathological processes in a better-differentiated way.

Keywords: objective measurement; cochlear implant; differential diagnostics

1. Introduction

Cochlear implantation is an established therapy for sensorineural hearing loss if hearing aids and other solutions fail to restore speech recognition [1,2]. Recent studies reported on successful cochlear implant (CI) provision for patients with hearing losses from 50 to 80 dB [3–6]. However, even in these patients, with good preconditions for postoperative word recognition—and even more in the established patient population with no preoperative word recognition [6]—some challenges still remain. Recent studies and opinions [3,7–10] indicate a lack of audiological differential diagnosis in these patients and highlight the observation that "the broad array of factors that contribute to speech recognition performance in adult CI users suggests the potential both for novel diagnostic assessment batteries to explain poor performance, and also new rehabilitation strategies for patients who exhibit poor outcomes" [7].

To our knowledge, there is no generally agreed classification of CI recipients with respect to performance or to speech perception in general. A prediction model recently introduced by Hoppe et al. [3] for the expected postoperative word recognition score at conversation level, WRS_{65}(CI), after six months of CI use would allow such a classification. Thus, failure to reach this goal can easily be assessed by routine clinical audiometry [3,6]. "Unexplained poor performance" may be defined as applying to CI recipients whose WRS_{65}(CI) does not meet the predicted score according to this model. Such cases can be observed with an incidence of around five percent in a population with residual preoperative word recognition score (WRS) [6] on the basis of a 20-percentage-points (pp) difference (WRS_{GAP}) between prediction and measurement in monosyllable test scores. Users who reach the predicted score later than six months after implantation (e.g., twelve months later) would not be covered by this definition [6]. More recently, in a study by Dziemba et al. [11] such a definition was applied in order to identify systematic differences in postoperative fitting of CI systems in a group of well and poorly performing CI recipients, namely the differences in audibility and the loudness growth function measured by categorical loudness scaling. An additional application of the prediction model [3] could be the interpretation of electrophysiological measurements based on prior classification of groups of recipients in respect of the WRS_{GAP}. Other recent work [8,12–15] led to the proposal and use of a setting for electrically evoked auditory brainstem responses (EABR) mimicking the established acoustic broadband click. Reference values for latencies were assessed by including only CI recipients with word recognition score with cochlear implant at 65 dB (WRS_{65}(CI)) of 50% or more [13]. This approach led to improved differential diagnosis for CI recipients and improved intraoperative assessment by using objective methods like electrically evoked compound action potentials (ECAP) and EABR [13,15,16].

Some characteristics of CI recipients, such as rate dependence of electrophysiological measurements, indicate a potential for improvement in differential diagnostics. In the acoustic modality, rate effects in auditory brainstem responses (ABR) are already well described [17,18]. Jiang et al. [18] reported age-dependent latencies and interpeak intervals in children as consequences of developmental effects. In our opinion, this measure of auditory synaptic efficacy [18] can be transferred to differential diagnostics in CI recipients to provide further explanation of unexpectedly poor WRS_{65}(CI) values. We expect that certain damage mechanisms in hearing-impaired subjects and CI recipients may have a similar effect on rate dependence of EABRs.

Consequently, the goal of this study was to provide reference values for rate-dependent EABR in CI recipients. By including only CI users who met the predicted values of WRS_{65}(CI), we aimed to open a window for differential diagnostics in CI recipients with unexpected and unexplained poor postoperative WRS_{65}(CI).

2. Materials and Methods

2.1. Research Subjects

This prospective investigation included five subjects in the pilot phase, and thereafter a further 20 subjects, according to a power calculation based on the results of the pilot phase. The power calculation was based on a effect size of 0.45 ms, which was the mean of the rate dependence of latency t5 of the pilot measurements (standard deviation of 0.22). We used a balanced one-way analysis of variance power calculation. The significance level was set to 0.05 and the power was set to 0.95.

The study was approved by the Ethics Committee at the University Medicine Greifswald on 10 August 2021 (BB 120/21), and all procedures were in accordance with the ethical standards of the institutional and national research committee and with the 1964 Helsinki declaration and its later amendments or comparable ethical standards. The study was registered in the German Clinical Trials Register (DRKS00026195 https://drks.de/search/de/trial/DRKS00026195 (accessed on 16 October 2023)).

Participants were recruited from the clinic's patient population. Inclusion criteria were:

- Adulthood (minimum age 18 years) at implantation;
- Implant type: CI24RE, CI400 series, CI500 series, or CI600 series (Cochlear™ Limited, Sydney, Australia);
- Implant in specification according to European Consensus Statement on Cochlear Implant Failures and Explantations [19];
- WRS_{65}(CI) in the upper three quartiles according to classification of Hoppe et al. [20];
- Willingness and ability to participate in the study.

Exclusion criteria were:

- Known mental handicap;
- Known central hearing disorders;
- Short cut or open circuit of intracochlear electrodes 11 and/or 18.

Demographic information for these patients is provided in Table 1. Bilateral implantation was not an exclusion criterion; in those two cases, both ears were included in the analysis separately (#098/#107 and #271/#275). The mean age at the time of inclusion in the study of the participants was 59 years (minimum age 38 years, maximum age 74 years). The participants had a mean hearing experience, usage of CI, of 51.4 months (min. = 1 month, max. = 146 months).

Table 1. Biographical data of participants.

ID	Age (Years)	Usage of CI (Months)	Side	Gender	Implant Type	Electrode Type	WRS_{65}(CI) (%)
#098	62	146	r	f	CI512	CA	75.0
#107	62	140	l	f	CI512	CA	85.0
#140	59	104	r	f	CI24RE	CA	92.5
#160	65	97	r	f	CI24RE	CA	67.5
#193	58	81	r	f	CI422	SS	75.0
#234	57	71	l	m	CI522	SS	55.0
#242	53	26	l	f	CI522	SS	87.5
#247	53	25	r	m	CI532	SM	85.0
#251	72	52	l	f	CI532	SM	75.0
#262	45	61	l	f	CI512	CA	75.0
#269	55	13	l	f	CI512	CA	77.5
#271	73	8	l	m	CI532	SM	80.0
#275	73	3	r	m	CI532	SM	60.0
#279	62	28	r	f	CI532	SM	82.5
#281	56	27	r	f	CI532	SM	87.5
#288	57	19	r	f	CI622	SS	82.5
#315	38	7	r	f	CI622	SS	75.0
#341	64	3	r	m	CI622	SS	87.5
#348	74	116	l	f	CI612	CA	82.5
#350	59	1	l	f	CI622	SS	60.0

'Age' is the recipient's age at the time of inclusion in the study. Side is coded right (r) or left (l) for ear receiving the implant. Recipient's sex is indicated, (f) or (m). Electrode types were: Contour Advance® (CA), Slim Modiolar (SM), and Slim Straight (SS).

2.2. Electrophysiological Measurements

To measure rate dependences of latencies and inter-peak latencies of EABRs, a quasi-simultaneous measurement of ECAPs and EABRs is needed. Here, it is essential to use the same stimulation mode and the same stimulation intensity for both assessments, to ensure compatibility of the data. Therefore, Dziemba et al. [12] introduced an intracochlear stimulation mode for the Nucleus® CI system ($EABR_{CI}$Stim). They used electrode 11 as a stimulation-active and electrode 18 as a stimulation-indifferent electrode, with a pulse width of 100 µs. This $EABR_{CI}$Stim facilitates an electrical excitation covering a median length of about 80% of the length of the implanted CI electrode array. Since ECAP and EABR are recorded with opposite polarity, the inter-peak latencies were determined between the negative peak of the ECAP and the corresponding positive peaks in the EABR, measured at the same stimulation intensity.

In order to avoid possible intensity-dependent effects, a defined supra-threshold stimulation intensity of 20 current levels (CLs) above the individual ECAP threshold, measured with the $EABR_{CI}$Stim, was set. The measurements in all subjects followed the same procedure, as described below.

2.2.1. ECAP Measurements

For the unconditional avoidance of uncomfortable loud stimulation the loudest acceptable presentation level (LAPL) using the $EABR_{CI}$Stim was estimated subjectively in a first step.

The second step was the identification of the most appropriate recording-active electrode according to Dziemba et al. [12]. Therefore, ECAP was measured at LAPL by stimulating all intra-cochlear electrodes, except electrodes 11 and 18, sequentially by using the extracochlear electrode (plate) MP2 as recording-indifferent electrode. The electrode with the largest ECAP amplitude at LAPL was selected as the best recording-active electrode.

In the third step, an ECAP amplitude-growth function was measured up to LAPL with the values found previously. The visual ECAP threshold was read out, taking into account a minimum signal-to-noise ratio for ECAP measurements according to Hey et al. [21].

Finally, the rate-dependent ECAPs were measured by using a stimulation intensity of 20 CL above the previously found threshold at stimulation rates of 11, 41, 81 and 91 stimuli per second.

2.2.2. EABR Measurements

All EABR measurement series were performed in the same stimulation mode as for the rate-dependent ECAP, using the $EABR_{CI}$Stim described above. The Eclipse system (Interacoustics, Middelfart, Denmark) was used to record the rate-dependent EABRs. Synchronisation between the CI system and the EABR device was achieved through a TTL-compatible trigger signal. This was sent via a commercially available cable (3.5 mm jack) from the programming interface of the CI system to the EABR recording system. The marking of all the measured potentials (ECAP and EABR) was performed according to Atcherson and Stoody [22]. To avoid ambivalence in picking peaks, they recommended that the rightmost sample be used for marking the positive peaks and the leftmost sample be used for marking the negative peaks. The labelling and numbering of the marked potentials was performed according to Jewett and Williston [23].

2.3. *Statistical Analysis*

We used boxplots, as defined by Tukey [24], for the graphical representation of the measured values.

For each user, the set of measurement data are a connected, non-normally distributed sample. Furthermore, there is no variance homogeneity of the data. Therefore, a non-parametric test must be used; we chose the Friedman rank sum test as being the most appropriate. As a post hocanalysis, we used the test of multiple comparison after Friedman test.

All statistical tests and figures were conducted with R [25] and RStudio [26].

3. Results

3.1. *Latencies*

The latencies t1, t3 and t5 of rate-dependent ECAP and EABR are shown in Figure 1. While no rate effect on latency t1 was seen for the ECAP ($p = 0.07$), we found significant mean rate effects for latency t3 (0.19 ms) and t5 (0.37 ms) The post hoc analyses of the rate effects of t3 and t5 are summarised in Tables 2 and 3.

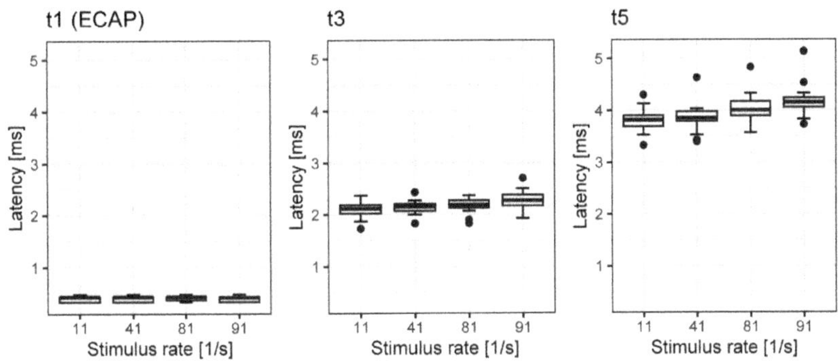

Figure 1. Latencies of all measured potentials. The boxes show medians and quartiles; the whiskers show the maximum value within 1.5 IQR (1.5 times the interquartile range). Filled circles show the outliers.

Table 2. Friedman rank sum test of latency t3 ($p = 2 \times 10^{-10}$), post hoc analysis.

	obs diff	critical diff	stat signif	p
11–41	13.5	21.5	FALSE	0.98
11–81	30.5	21.5	TRUE	0.001
11–91	52.0	21.5	TRUE	2×10^{-9}
41–81	17.0	21.5	FALSE	0.37
41–91	38.5	21.5	TRUE	2×10^{-5}
81–91	21.5	21.5	FALSE	0.08

Table 3. Friedman rank sum test of latency t5 ($p = 3 \times 10^{-10}$), post hoc analysis.

	obs diff	critical diff	stat signif	p
11–41	4.0	21.5	FALSE	1.0
11–81	29.5	21.5	TRUE	0.003
11–91	48.5	21.5	TRUE	3×10^{-8}
41–81	25.5	21.5	TRUE	0.02
41–91	44.5	21.5	TRUE	5×10^{-7}
81–91	19.0	21.5	FALSE	0.19

3.2. Interpeak Intervals

The interpeak intervals t5 − t1, t5 − t3 and t3 − t1 of rate-dependent ECAPs and EABRs are shown in Figure 2. We found significant rate effects for all the interpeak intervals analysed. The interpeak interval t5 − t1 shows a rate effect of 0.37 ms, while the interpeak interval t5 − t3 is shows a rate effect of 0.18 ms. The mean rate effect on interpeak interval t3 − t1 is 0.19 ms. The analyses are summarised in Tables 4–6.

Table 4. Friedman rank sum test of t5 − t1 interpeak interval ($p = 3 \times 10^{-10}$), post hoc analysis.

	obs diff	critical diff	stat signif	p
11–41	4.0	21.5	FALSE	1.0
11–81	29.5	21.5	TRUE	0.003
11–91	48.5	21.5	TRUE	3×10^{-8}
41–81	25.5	21.5	TRUE	0.02
41–91	44.5	21.5	TRUE	5×10^{-7}
81–91	19.0	21.5	FALSE	0.20

Table 5. Friedman rank sum test of t5 − t3 interpeak interval ($p = 1 \times 10^{-8}$), post hoc analysis.

	obs diff	critical diff	stat signif	p
11–41	3.5	21.5	FALSE	1.0
11–81	29.5	21.5	TRUE	0.003
11–91	38.0	21.5	TRUE	3×10^{-5}
41–81	33.0	21.5	TRUE	5×10^{-4}
41–91	41.5	21.5	TRUE	4×10^{-6}
81–91	8.5	21.5	FALSE	1.0

Table 6. Friedman rank sum test of t3 − t1 interpeak interval ($p = 2 \times 10^{-10}$), post hoc analysis.

	obs diff	critical diff	stat signif	p
11–41	13.5	21.5	FALSE	0.99
11–81	30.5	21.5	TRUE	0.002
11–91	52.0	21.5	TRUE	2×10^{-9}
41–81	17.0	21.5	FALSE	0.37
41–91	38.5	21.5	TRUE	2×10^{-5}
81–91	21.5	21.5	FALSE	0.08

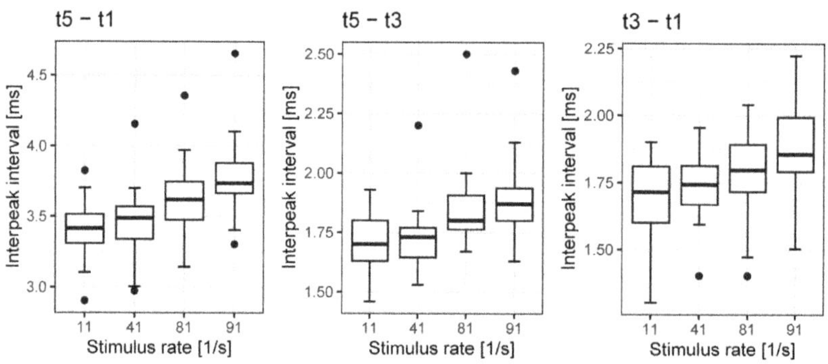

Figure 2. Interpeak intervals of all measured potentials. The boxes show medians and quartiles; the whiskers show the maximum value within 1.5 IQR. Filled circles show the outliers.

3.3. Amplitudes

The amplitudes A1, A3 and A5 of rate-dependent ECAPs and EABRs are shown in Figure 3. While for ECAP, there is no rate effect on A1 ($p = 0.26$), we found significant detrimental rate effects, for A3 and A5, with respective mean reductions of 73% and 81%. The post hoc analyses of the rate effects of A3 and A5 are summarised in Tables 7 and 8.

Table 7. Friedman rank sum test of amplitude A3 ($p = 9 \times 10^{-5}$), post hoc analysis.

	obs diff	critical diff	stat signif	p
11–41	2.0	21.5	FALSE	1.0
11–81	21.0	21.5	FALSE	0.10
11–91	29.0	21.5	TRUE	0.004
41–81	23.0	21.5	TRUE	0.048
41–91	31.0	21.5	TRUE	0.001
81–91	8.0	21.5	FALSE	1.0

Table 8. Friedman rank sum test of amplitude A5 ($p = 2 \times 10^{-5}$), post hoc analysis.

	obs diff	critical diff	stat signif	p
11–41	16.0	21.5	FALSE	0.50
11–81	17.0	21.5	FALSE	0.37
11–91	19.0	21.5	FALSE	0.20
41–81	33.0	21.5	TRUE	5×10^{-4}
41–91	35.0	21.5	TRUE	2×10^{-4}
81–91	2.0	21.5	FALSE	1.0

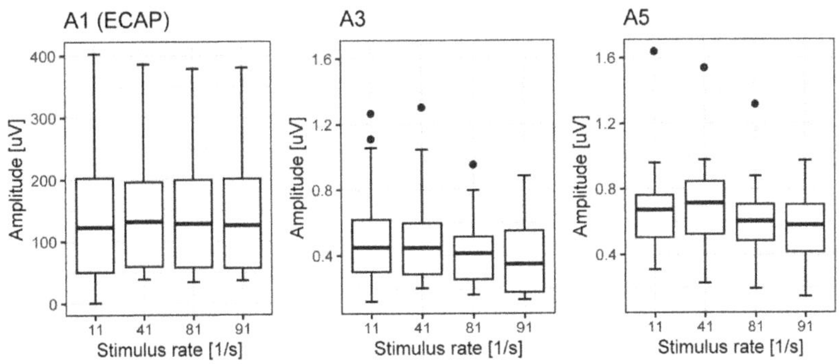

Figure 3. Amplitudes of all measured potentials. The boxes show medians and quartiles; the whiskers show the maximum value within 1.5 IQR. Filled circles show the outliers.

4. Discussion

In accordance with the study's goals, we investigated the rate dependences in our population of CI recipients, all of whom had monosyllabic word recognition within the upper three quartiles according to the classification put forward by Hoppe et al. [20]. We found rate dependences for EABR latency t3 and t5 in the order of 0.19 ms and 0.37 ms, respectively, while ECAPs were not affected by rate. Correspondingly, the interpeak intervals' rate dependences for t5 − t1, t5 − t3 and t3 − t1 were found to be in the order of 0.37 ms, 0.18 ms and 0.19 ms. Jiang et al. [18] described the change in rate dependence in acoustic ABR as an effect of the maturing auditory pathway in children of various ages. In adults, the latency changes with rate are probably related to synaptic adaptation [17]. With respect to the amplitudes, Campbell et al. [27] have stated that the change in wave V of acoustic ABR does not decrease at 81/s by more than 28% compared with the amplitude at 11/s. However, in our population, we found significant detrimental rate effects: a reduction down to 73% for A3 and down to 81% for A5. This is within the range for rate-dependent changes found for wave V in acoustic ABR [27]. To summarise, these reference values for EABR and ECAP latencies, interpeak intervals and amplitudes provide a basis for possible differential diagnoses after cochlear implantation.

We hypothesize that in postlingually deafened adults with CI, larger changes in amplitudes and latencies due to rate (in comparison with references values) can be interpreted as pathological effects. The values shown above can be regarded as reference values. Pathologies may then be revealed in significant deviations from them. For example, in patients with auditory neuropathy spectrum disorder the dyssynchronous neural activity may affect temporal encoding of electrical stimulation from a cochlear implant [28]. Even though Fulmer et al. [28] investigated the recovery function of ECAP, one may reasonably assume that EABR measurements and their rate dependences will be affected by these pathological mechanisms as well. Continuing this line of thought, we would argue that, compared with ECAP, EABR assesses the higher levels of the auditory pathway as well, and therefore appears to offer a valuable complement within differential diagnostics. However, while ECAP can be considered to provide tonotopic information, the EABR as applied in this study will provide integrated information about the status of the auditory pathway. This differential diagnostic pattern is especially important for the most recent CI population [3–6] with higher preoperative speech recognition scores. In this patient population, a highly predictive outcome was observed [3,6] compared with the established patient population with no preoperative speech perception [6,29]

Consequently, if in the patient population with good audiometric preoperative conditions [6] the prediction cannot be achieved, an underlying pathology of the auditory pathway may be suspected. Moreover, approaches utilising advanced measurements of ECAPs [8,30–33], and the assessment of EABR and its rate dependences might be suitable in analogy to the findings in acoustic ABR. With values up to 0.28 ms the standard deviation for the interpeak interval $t5 - t1$ seems to be slightly higher than the 0.23 ms found by Campbell et al. [27]. A more thorough analysis will be needed in future studies.

Assuming a higher standard deviation (which still has to be confirmed), this may have its root cause in the inclusion criteria of the CI population. For acoustic stimulation, normative values, and the population in which to assess them, are easy to define as one has by definition to include normal-hearing subjects. In the case of CI recipients, the definition of a reference group is far more challenging. There are no generally agreed criteria for the derivation of a reference group. Consequently, the reference values provided by this study can potentially be improved by better outcome prediction models and, based on this, a narrower patient selection.

Recently, Hoppe et al. [6] applied the criterion "unexpectedly poor speech perception", defined as monosyllabic speech recognition $\geq$ 20 pp lower than predicted after six months, in order to discuss the time course of such cases. The six months were derived from study which found that 90% of the final score is achieved after 6.9 months. Even if in that study [6] the majority of subjects who were poor perfomers after six months nonetheless reached the target value after a longer time period, there remain 5% of cases in which the prediction is not reached in the long run. The aim of differential diagnostics using EABR would be to differentiate between a patient's intrinsic root causes for unexpectedly poor speech perception (pathologies) or causes in which the fitting of CI system also plays a part [11]. Future studies with a focus on the time course of postoperative speech recognition with respect to different pathologies (once these are confirmed) will be needed to refine the diagnostics using EABR.

5. Conclusions

The rate-dependences of latency and amplitude in EABR have characteristics comparable to those of acoustic ABR. Consequently, EABR may potentially support differential diagnosis in CI recipients with an outcome below expectation. The results of this study may serve to provide reference values. Pathological issues of the peripheral auditory pathway hindering a postoperative increase in speech perception and CI outcome in general can be excluded or confirmed.

Author Contributions: Conceptualization, O.C.D.; methodology, O.C.D., T.H. and F.I.; software, O.C.D.; validation, O.C.D.; formal analysis, O.C.D.; investigation, O.C.D.; resources, O.C.D., T.B., T.H. and F.I.; data curation, O.C.D.; writing—original draft preparation, O.C.D. and T.H.; writing—review and editing, O.C.D., F.I. and T.B.; visualization, O.C.D.; supervision, F.I.; project administration, O.C.D. and T.H.; funding acquisition, O.C.D. All authors have read and agreed to the published version of the manuscript.

Funding: This research was funded by Cochlear™ Research an Development Limited grant number IIR-2311.

Institutional Review Board Statement: Ethical approval by Ethics Committee at the University Medicine Greifswald. Approval code: BB 120/21 Approval date: 10 August 2021. This study was registered in German Clinical Trials Register under DRKS-ID: DRKS00026195 https://drks.de/search/de/trial/DRKS00026195 (accessed on 16 October 2023).

Informed Consent Statement: Informed consent was obtained from all subjects involved in the study.

Data Availability Statement: The data presented in this study are available on request from the corresponding author. The data are not publicly available due to data protection regulations.

Conflicts of Interest: O.D. received funding in other projects and travel money. T.H. is employee of Cochlear Deutschland GmbH & Co. KG. T.B. and F.I. declare no conflict of interest.

Abbreviations

ABR	auditory brainstem responses
CI	cochlear implant
CL	current level
critical diff	critical differences
EABR	electrically evoked auditory brainstem responses
ECAP	electrically evoked compound action potentials
$EABR_{CI}Stim$	EABR stimulation mode according to [12]
IQR	interquartile range
LAPL	loudest acceptable presentation level
obs diff	observed differences
pp	percentage-points
stat signif	statistical significance (boolean value)
WRS	word recognition score
$WRS_{65}(CI)$	word recognition score with cochlear implant at 65 dB

References

1. Buchman, C.A.; Gifford, R.H.; Haynes, D.S.; Lenarz, T.; O'Donoghue, G.; Adunka, O.; Biever, A.; Briggs, R.J.; Carlson, M.L.; Dai, P.; et al. Unilateral Cochlear Implants for Severe, Profound, or Moderate Sloping to Profound Bilateral Sensorineural Hearing Loss: A Systematic Review and Consensus Statements. *JAMA Otolaryngol. Head Neck Surg.* **2020**, *146*, 942–953. [CrossRef][PubMed]
2. Deutsche Gesellschaft für Hals-Nasen-Ohren-Heilkunde, Kopf- und Hals-Chirurgie e.V. S2k-Leitlinie Cochlea-Implantat Versorgung, Version 3.0. 31 October 2020. Available online: https://register.awmf.org/de/leitlinien/detail/017-071 (accessed on 16 October 2023).
3. Hoppe, U.; Hocke, T.; Hast, A.; Iro, H. Cochlear Implantation in Candidates with Moderate-to-Severe Hearing Loss and Poor Speech Perception. *Laryngoscope* **2021**, *131*, E940–E945. [CrossRef] [PubMed]
4. Thangavelu, K.; Nitzge, M.; Weiß, R.M.; Mueller-Mazzotta, J.; Stuck, B.A.; Reimann, K. Role of cochlear reserve in adults with cochlear implants following post-lingual hearing loss. *Eur. Arch. Oto-Rhino Head Neck* **2023**, *280*, 1063–1071. [CrossRef] [PubMed]
5. Rieck, J.H.; Beyer, A.; Mewes, A.; Caliebe, A.; Hey, M. Extended Preoperative Audiometry for Outcome Prediction and Risk Analysis in Patients Receiving Cochlear Implants. *J. Clin. Med.* **2023**, *12*, 3262. [CrossRef] [PubMed]
6. Hoppe, U.; Hast, A.; Hocke, T. Validation of a predictive model for speech discrimination after cochlear implant provision. *HNO* **2023**, *71*, 53–59. [CrossRef]
7. Moberly, A.C.; Bates, C.; Harris, M.S.; Pisoni, D.B. The Enigma of Poor Performance by Adults with Cochlear Implants. *Otol. Neurotol.* **2016**, *37*, 1522–1528. [CrossRef] [PubMed]
8. Hoth, S.; Dziemba, O.C. The role of auditory evoked potentials in the context of cochlear implant provision: Presented at the Annual Meeting of ADANO 2015 in Bern. *Otol. Neurotol.* **2017**, *38*, e522–e530. [CrossRef]
9. Peter, M.S.; Warnecke, A.; Staecker, H. A Window of Opportunity: Perilymph Sampling from the Round Window Membrane Can Advance Inner Ear Diagnostics and Therapeutics. *J. Clin. Med.* **2022**, *11*, 316. [CrossRef]
10. Yawn, R.J.; Nassiri, A.M.; Rivas, A. Auditory Neuropathy: Bridging the Gap Between Hearing Aids and Cochlear Implants. *Otolaryngol. Clin. N. Am.* **2019**, *52*, 349–355. [CrossRef]
11. Dziemba, O.C.; Merz, S.; Hocke, T. Zur evaluierenden Audiometrie nach Cochlea-Implantat-Versorgung. *HNO* **2023**, *71*, 669–677. [CrossRef]
12. Dziemba, O.C.; Hocke, T.; Müller, A.; Kaftan, H. Excitation characteristic of a bipolar stimulus for broadband stimulation in measurements of electrically evoked auditory potentials. *Z. Für Med. Phys.* **2018**, *28*, 73–77. [CrossRef]
13. Dziemba, O.C.; Hocke, T.; Müller, A. EABR on cochlear implant—Measurements from clinical routine compared to reference values. *GMS Z. Für Audiol. Audiol. Acoust.* **2022**, *4*. [CrossRef]
14. Holtmann, L.C.; Strahlenbach, A.; Hans, S.; Lang, S.; Arweiler-Harbeck, D. Visualizing Contralateral Suppression of Hearing Sensitivity via Acoustic and Electric Brainstem Audiometry in Bimodal Cochlear Implant Patients: A Feasibility Study. *Audiol. Neurotol.* **2022**, *28*, 158–168. [CrossRef]
15. Rahne, T.; Hocke, T.; Strauß, C.; Kösling, S.; Fröhlich, L.; Plontke, S.K. Perioperative Recording of Cochlear Implant Evoked Brain Stem Responses after Removal of the Intralabyrinthine Portion of a Vestibular Schwannoma in a Patient with NF2. *Otol. Neurotol.* **2019**, *40*, e20–e24. [CrossRef] [PubMed]

16. Müller, A.; Feick, J.; Dziemba, O.C.; Mir-Salim, P. Objective Diagnostics and Therapie of Hearing Loss Several Years after Cochlear Implant. *Laryngo-Rhino-Otologie* **2016**, *95*, 634–635. [CrossRef] [PubMed]
17. Picton, T.W. *Human Auditory Evoked Potentials;* Plural Publishing: San Diego, CA, USA, 2010.
18. Jiang, Z.D.; Wu, Y.Y.; Zheng, W.S.; Sun, D.K.; Feng, L.Y.; Liu, X.Y. The effect of click rate on latency and interpeak interval of the brain-stem auditory evoked potentials in children from birth to 6 years. *Electroencephalogr. Clin. Neurophysiol.* **1991**, *80*, 60–64. [CrossRef] [PubMed]
19. European Consensus Statement on Cochlear Implant Failures and Explantations: Editorial. *Otol. Neurotol.* **2005**, *26*, 1097–1099. [CrossRef]
20. Hoppe, U.; Hocke, T.; Hast, A.; Iro, H. Maximum preimplantation monosyllabic score as predictor of cochlear implant outcome. *HNO* **2019**, *62*, 62–68. [CrossRef]
21. Hey, M.; Müller-Deile, J. Accuracy of measurement in electrically evoked compound action potentials. *J. Neurosci. Methods* **2015**, *239*, 214–222. [CrossRef]
22. Atcherson, S.R.; Stoody, T.M. (Eds.) Chapter 3: Principles of Analysis an Interpretation. In *Auditory Electrophysiology;* Thieme: New York, NY, USA, 2012; pp. 27–40.
23. Jewett, D.L.; Williston, J.S. Auditory-evoked far fields averaged from the scalp of humans. *Brain* **1971**, *94*, 681–696. [CrossRef]
24. Tukey, J.W. *Exploratory Data Analysis;* Addison-Wesley Publishing Company: Reading, MA, USA, 1977.
25. R Core Team. *R: A Language and Environment for Statistical Computing;* R Foundation for Statistical Computing: Vienna, Austria, 2021.
26. Posit Team. *RStudio: Integrated Development Environment for R;* Posit Software, PBC: Boston, MA, USA, 2023. Available online: http://www.posit.co/ (accessed on 16 October 2023).
27. Campbell, K.B.; Picton, T.W.; Wolfe, R.G.; Maru, J.; Baribeau-Braun, J.; Braun, C. Auditory Potentials. *Sensus* **1981**, *1*, 21–31.
28. Fulmer, S.L.; Runge, C.L.; Jensen, J.W.; Friedland, D.R. Rate of neural recovery in implanted children with auditory neuropathy spectrum disorder. *Otolaryngol. Head Neck Surg.* **2011**, *144*, 274–279. [CrossRef] [PubMed]
29. Shafieibavani, E.; Goudey, B.; Kiral, I.; Zhong, P.; Jimeno-Yepes, A.; Swan, A.; Gambhir, M.; Buechner, A.; Kludt, E.; Eikelboom, R.H.; et al. Predictive models for cochlear implant outcomes: Performance, generalizability, and the impact of cohort size. *Trends Hear.* **2021**, *25*, 23312165211066174. [CrossRef] [PubMed]
30. Botros, A.; Psarros, C. Neural Response Telemetry Reconsidered: II. The Influence of Neural Population on the ECAP Recovery Function and Refractoriness. *Ear Hear.* **2010**, *31*, 380–391. [CrossRef] [PubMed]
31. Dong, Y.; Briaire, J.J.; Stronks, H.C.; Frijns, J.H.M. Speech Perception Performance in Cochlear Implant Recipients Correlates to the Number and Synchrony of Excited Auditory Nerve Fibers Derived from Electrically Evoked Compound Action Potentials. *Ear Hear.* **2023**, *44*, 276–286. [CrossRef] [PubMed]
32. Garcia, C.; Goehring, T.; Cosentino, S.; Turner, R.E.; Deeks, J.M.; Brochier, T.; Rughooputh, T.; Bance, M.; Carlyon, R.P. The Panoramic ECAP Method: Estimating Patient-Specific Patterns of Current Spread and Neural Health in Cochlear Implant Users. *J. Assoc. Res. Otolaryngol.* **2021**, *22*, 567–589. [CrossRef] [PubMed]
33. He, S.; Abbas, P.J.; Doyle, D.V.; McFayden, T.C.; Mulherin, S. Temporal Response Properties of the Auditory Nerve in Implanted Children with Auditory Neuropathy Spectrum Disorder and Implanted Children with Sensorineural Hearing Loss. *Ear Hear.* **2016**, *37*, 397–411. [CrossRef]

Journal of
Clinical Medicine

MDPI

Article

Investigation of Maximum Monosyllabic Word Recognition as a Predictor of Speech Understanding with Cochlear Implant

Ronja Czurda [1,*], Thomas Wesarg [1], Antje Aschendorff [1], Rainer Linus Beck [1], Thomas Hocke [2], Manuel Christoph Ketterer [1] and Susan Arndt [1]

[1] Department of Otorhinolaryngology, Medical Center—University of Freiburg, Faculty of Medicine, University of Freiburg, Killianstr. 5, 79106 Freiburg, Germany; thomas.wesarg@uniklinik-freiburg.de (T.W.); antje.aschendorff@uniklinik-freiburg.de (A.A.); rainer.beck@uniklinik-freiburg.de (R.L.B.); manuel.christoph.ketterer@uniklinik-freiburg.de (M.C.K.); susan.arndt@uniklinik-freiburg.de (S.A.)

[2] Cochlear Deutschland GmbH & Co., KG, Mailänder Straße 4 a, 30539 Hannover, Germany; thocke@cochlear.com

* Correspondence: ronja.czurda@uniklinik-freiburg.de

Abstract: Background: The cochlear implant (CI) is an established treatment option for patients with inadequate speech understanding and insufficient aided scores. Nevertheless, reliable predictive models and specific therapy goals regarding achievable speech understanding are still lacking. **Method:** In this retrospective study, 601 cases of CI fittings between 2005 and 2021 at the University Medical Center Freiburg were analyzed. We investigated the preoperative unaided maximum word recognition score (mWRS) as a minimum predictor for post-interventional scores at 65 dB SPL, WRS_{65}(CI). The WRS_{65}(CI) was compared with the preoperative-aided WRS, and a previously published prediction model for the WRS_{65}(CI) was reviewed. Furthermore, the effect of duration of hearing loss, duration of HA fitting, and etiology on WRS_{65}(CI) were investigated. **Results:** In 95.5% of the cases, a significant improvement in word recognition was observed after CI. WRS_{65}(CI) achieved or exceeded mWRS in 97% of cases. Etiology had a significant impact on WRS_{65}(CI). The predicted score was missed by more than 20 percentage points in 12.8% of cases. **Discussion:** Our results confirmed the minimum prediction via mWRS. A more precise prediction of the expected WRS_{65}(CI) is possible. The etiology of hearing loss should be considered in the indication and postoperative care to achieve optimal results.

Keywords: cochlear implant; speech audiometry; word recognition; hearing loss; hearing aid; maximum word recognition

1. Introduction

In recent decades, the cochlear implant (CI) has become an established treatment option for patients with severe to profound hearing loss or impairment, for whom the fitting of a hearing aid (HA) or other hearing amplification measures no longer ensure adequate speech understanding [1–5]. Progressive improvements in surgery, technology, and rehabilitation measures have led to a constant expansion of the indication criteria [6–11], so that, since 2020, the S2k guideline in Germany recommends cochlear implantation of a patient from the point of monosyllabic word recognition of ≤60% at a sound level of 65 dB SPL after optimized HA fitting [2]. This specific value for the audiological indication has not yet been matched by a value of speech understanding that should be achieved postoperatively in German-speaking countries. According to the guidelines for cochlear implant treatment of the German Society of Oto-Rhino-Laryngology, an improvement in speech understanding of at least 20 percentage points with cochlear implantation can be expected [5]. In addition, initial studies highlight preoperative maximum word recognition (mWRS) as a suitable individual predictor for postoperative word recognition with CI at 65 dB SPL [12–14], referred to as WRS_{65}(CI) in the following. In the typical German clinic population of the last decade, approximately 96% of patients can be assumed to have a WRS_{65}(CI) that achieved or exceeded the preoperative mWRS [12].

Model approaches are available for the expected outcomes of care, which appear suitable for determining an expectation corridor for a patient population [15,16], which aims to provide individual predictions of expected postoperative WRS [17,18]. Hoppe et al. [17] have so far achieved a prediction error in the order of 11–14 percentage points (pp) with their model for sample sizes of about 100 patients with preoperatively measurable mWRS [19]. In this model, mWRS, monosyllabic word recognition with a HA at 65 dB SPL, WRS_{65}(HA), and the patient's age at the time of CI surgery are taken into account according to Equation (1):

$$WRS_{65}(CI)\ [\%] = \frac{100}{1 + e^{-(ß_0 + ß_1 \cdot mWRS + ß_2 \cdot Age + ß_3 \cdot WRS_{65}(HA))}} \quad (1)$$

where $ß_0 = 0.84 \pm 0.18$, $ß_1 = (0.012 \pm 0.0015)/\%$, $ß_2 = (-0.0094 \pm 0.0025)/\text{years}$, and $ß_3 = (0.0059 \pm 0.0026)/\%$.

However, this prediction is limited to patients with a preoperative mWRS greater than zero [19]. Until now, factors such as etiology, duration of hearing loss, duration of HA use, and duration of untreated hearing loss have not been taken into account in relation to the equation, and insufficient case numbers have also been problematic [17,19].

The aim of this study was to evaluate both approaches: the minimum prediction of the WRS_{65}(CI) based on the mWRS [12] and the model according to Equation (1). Both result "in a corridor within which the postoperative word recognition score with CI should be" [19], in the largest group of patients (to our knowledge) with a mWRS greater than 0%. The influence of etiology, duration of hearing loss, and duration of HA fitting on WRS_{65}(CI) and the deviation from the prognosis according to Equation (1) was additionally investigated.

2. Materials and Methods

The present retrospective study was performed with the approval of the Ethics Committee Freiburg (EK-Freiburg: 23-1029-S1-retro) (DRKS00029966) and in compliance with national law and the Declaration of Helsinki of 2013 (in the current revised edition).

2.1. Patients

The present data were collected between January 2005 and December 2021 within the framework of CI pre-evaluation and during basic and follow-up therapies of CI care in the Department of Otolaryngology at the University Medical Center Freiburg. The inclusion criteria were defined as uni- or bilateral implantation, age over 18 years at the time of implantation, measurable preoperative unaided monosyllabic word recognition in the implanted ear greater than 0%, together with available data on preoperative speech understanding with HA, CI experience of at least 6 months, and completed CI rehabilitation in Freiburg. Data from patients with neurological or psychiatric concomitant diseases relevant to speech understanding were excluded. Medical history data included age, gender, duration of subjective hearing loss, and etiology.

A total of 601 ears (cases) from 531 patients, 70 of whom were fitted bilaterally with CI, were identified to meet the inclusion criteria and were included. The demographic distribution of this study population is summarized in Table 1. The information on the duration of hearing loss and HA usage was collected through a questionnaire and is based on the subjective assessment of the patients. Figure 1 presents the distribution of etiologies of hearing loss. The "childhood disease" category includes mumps, measles, and rubella. Causes such as acoustic neuroma, medulloblastoma, and superficial siderosis have been grouped into cerebral diseases.

Table 1. Demographics of the patient population.

	Male Ears	Female Ears	
Sex	271	330	
Mean age at cochlear implantation [years]	56.2	51.4	
	Mean value	Standard deviation	
Duration of hearing loss [years]	26.3	16.9	
Presumed duration of hearing aid fitting [years]	20.4	14.1	
Implant side	Right	Left	
	290	311	
	Yes	No	Unknown
Tinnitus	363	214	24
Vestibulopathies	98	477	26

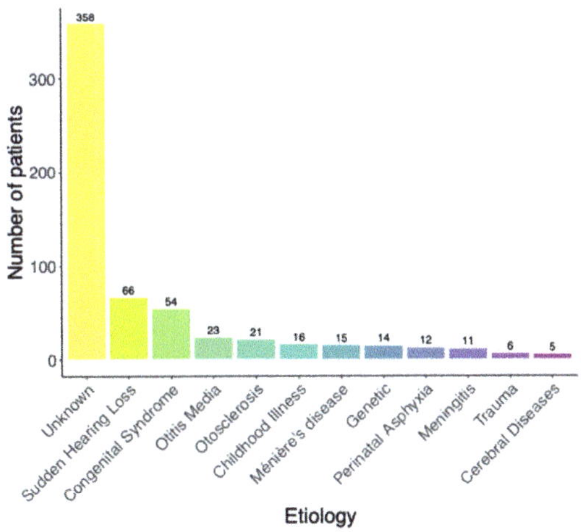

Figure 1. Distribution of etiologies of hearing loss.

2.2. Audiometry

Hearing loss in air conduction was averaged over the four octave frequencies (500, 1000, 2000, and 4000 Hz) and is reported here as a four-frequency-pure tone average (4PTA). The hearing thresholds were measured with headphones in a soundproof room for each ear separately. The opposite ear was masked, if necessary. For hearing thresholds exceeding the performance limit of the audiometers, a value of 120 dB HL was used in the analysis.

Speech understanding was assessed as word recognition in silence using the Freiburg monosyllabic test. Preoperatively, the mWRS and the WRS_{65}(HA) were measured. Postoperatively, the WRS_{65}(CI) was assessed after a period of at least six months after initial fitting.

2.3. Data Analysis

The statistical analysis of the data and the creation of the figures were carried out with R (R version 4.2.1; R Core Team (2023). R: A language and environment for statistical computing. R Foundation for Statistical Computing, Vienna, URL. https://www.R-project.org/ accessed on 15 February 2023).

To check for a normal distribution, the data sets were assessed using a Q-Q plot.

We performed statistical analysis to investigate the impact of (1) duration of hearing loss and (2) etiology.

(1) To investigate the impact of duration on hearing loss, we applied unpaired *t*-tests. Using the unpaired *t*-test, we compare the mean values of WRS_{65}(CI) between the group with a hearing loss > 20 years and the group with a hearing loss $\leq$ 20 years.
(2) The effect of etiology on WRS_{65}(CI) was analysed using a Kruskal–Wallis test. To further investigate the impact of etiology on postoperative outcome, post hoc comparisons were made between the various causes of severe to profound hearing loss using Dunn's test. To correct for multiple testing, a Holm adjustment was applied.

Missing data were not imputed. Cases with missing preoperative aided scores were excluded from model calculations according to Equation (1) but used for the evaluation of the minimum prediction via mWRS.

3. Results

3.1. Preoperative Results

Figure 2 illustrates the distribution of the duration of hearing loss and age at cochlear implantation and the duration of unaided hearing loss [duration of hearing loss − duration of hearing aid fitting]. The duration of hearing loss was defined retrospectively as the duration between the anamnestic onset and the time of the preoperative assessment of this loss.

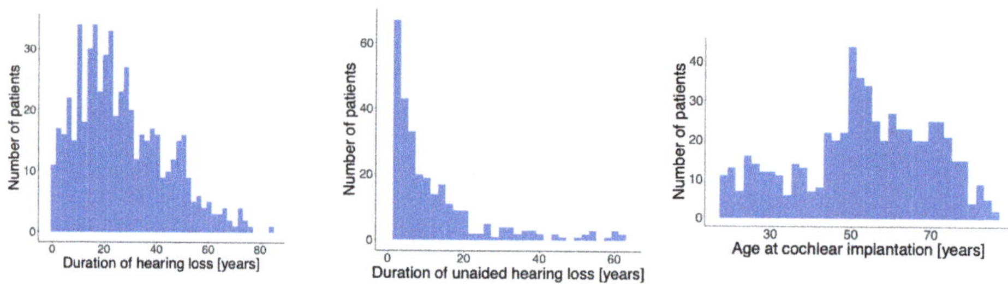

(a) (b) (c)

Figure 2. Patient characteristics. (**a**) Distribution of duration of hearing loss. (**b**) Distribution of duration of unaided hearing loss. (**c**) Distribution of age at cochlear implantation.

On average, patients reported a duration of hearing loss of 26.3 ± 17.0 years and a duration of HA fitting of 20.4 ± 14 years. Data were missing in 62 cases.

Based on the calculation of the duration of unaided hearing loss, an unaided period of >10 years was determined for 111 ears. Of these, 46 cases had unaided hearing loss for more than 20 years.

On average, the cases with unaided hearing loss for >20 years (n = 46) achieved a mean WRS_{65}(CI) of 68.6% ± 25.0%, whereas the cohort with untreated hearing loss for $\leq$20 years (n = 493 cases) achieved 74.2% ± 20.4%. The WRS_{65}(CI) was 74.0% ± 21.0% for the entire study population (n = 601).

(1) Applying an unpaired *t*-test between subjects with a duration of hearing loss >20 years and those with $\leq$20 years, we found no significant difference in the WRS_{65}(CI) ($p > 0.05$).

Figure 3 illustrates the relationships between different preoperative measurements. Figure 3a shows the relationship between the 4PTA and the mWRS. Overall, 43 ears (7.2%) had a 4PTA of <70 dB HL. Among these, 20 ears (3.3%) only achieved an mWRS of $\leq$50%, despite showing a low 4PTA. One hundred ears showed a 4PTA between 70 and 80 dB HL, 144 between 80 and 90 dB HL, and 308 greater than 90 dB. In five cases, these measurements are missing. Figure 3b shows the WRS_{65}(HA) versus the 4PTA, whereas Figure 3c plots the WRS_{65}(HA) versus the mWRS.

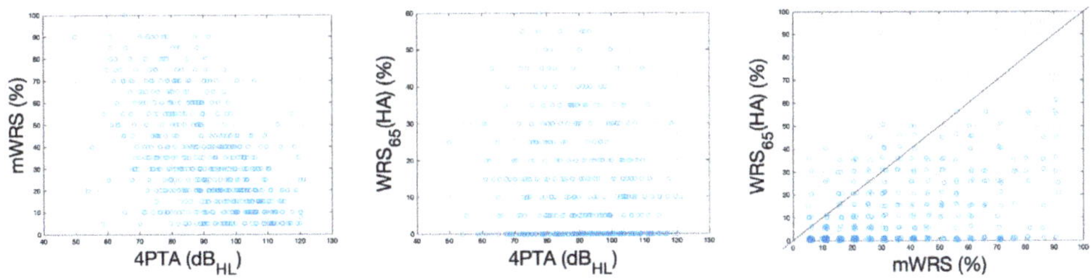

(a) (b) (c)

Figure 3. Scatterplots of pre- and postoperative word recognition in relation to different preoperative measurements. (**a**) Four-frequency pure-tone average, 4PTA, versus mWRS; (**b**) 4PTA versus WRS_{65}(HA). (**c**) Preoperative mWRS versus WRS_{65}(HA). The boundaries around the bisectors represent the critical differences, according to Winkler and Holube [20]. Points outside these limits can be interpreted as significant differences in the respective values.

The group results of the preoperative measurements are illustrated in Table 2.

Table 2. Preoperative four-frequency pure-tone average, 4PTA, and pre- and postoperative word recognition scores.

Preoperative	Minimum	Maximum	Mean	Standard Deviation
4PTA (dB HL)	49.8	120.0	91.0	14.2
mWRS (%)	5.0	100.0	33.2	22.6
WRS_{65}(HA) (%)	0.0	60.0	10.4	14.2

3.2. Postoperative Results

Figure 4a shows the relationship between the WRS_{65}(CI) and the preoperative 4PTA, whereas Figure 4b relates the WRS_{65}(CI) to the WRS_{65}(HA). Figure 4c presents the relationship between the postoperative WRS_{65}(CI) and the preoperative mWRS.

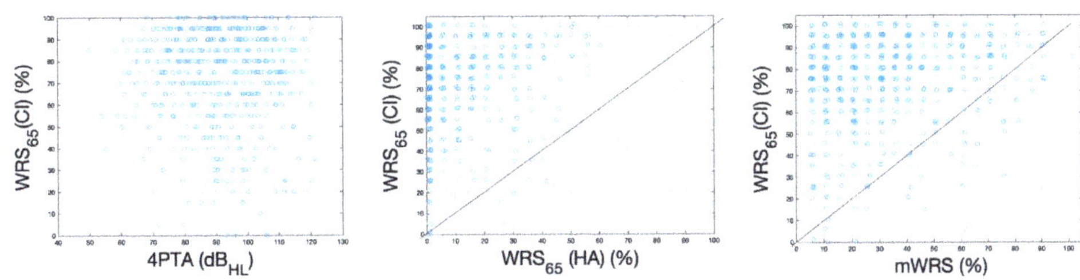

(a) (b) (c)

Figure 4. Scatterplots of postoperative word recognition in relation to preoperative measurements. (**a**) Postoperative WRS_{65}(CI) versus preoperative four-frequency pure-tone average, 4PTA. (**b**) WRS_{65}(CI) versus preoperative WRS_{65}(HA). (**c**) WRS_{65}(CI) versus preoperative mWRS. The boundaries around the bisectors represent the critical differences, according to Winkler and Holube [20]. Points outside these limits can be interpreted as significant differences in the respective values.

Until 2012, it was standard practice in our clinics, as in many other clinics in Germany, to measure monosyllabic word recognition with a HA at 70 dB SPL because of the otherwise often lack of speech recognition at lower sound pressure levels. Therefore, data concerning monosyllabic word recognition at 65 dB SPL with a HA were only available for 494 ears. Of these, 95.5% (n = 472) ears showed significantly improved word recognition with CI compared to word recognition with HA, both at 65 dB SPL. A significant deterioration [20] was only observed in one case (Figure 4b). The average speech understanding increases overall from an WRS_{65}(HA) of 10% to an WRS_{65}(CI) of 74%/65 dB. This corresponds to an improvement of 74%.

The scatterplot of the mWRS and the WRS_{65}(CI) in Figure 4c shows that the mWRS was achieved or exceeded by the WRS_{65}(CI) in 97% (n = 582) of cases. Thus, only 3% (n = 19) of cases yielded a WRS_{65}(CI) below the minimum predictor for the outcome with CI.

3.3. Effect of Etiology on Postoperative Speech Understanding

Figure 5 shows box-whisker plots of word recognition with CI for the different etiologies of hearing loss. In the comparisons of WRS_{65}(CI) between the different etiologies, the group with an unknown cause of deafness was excluded from the analysis in order to identify specific and clinically relevant differences between the known etiologies.

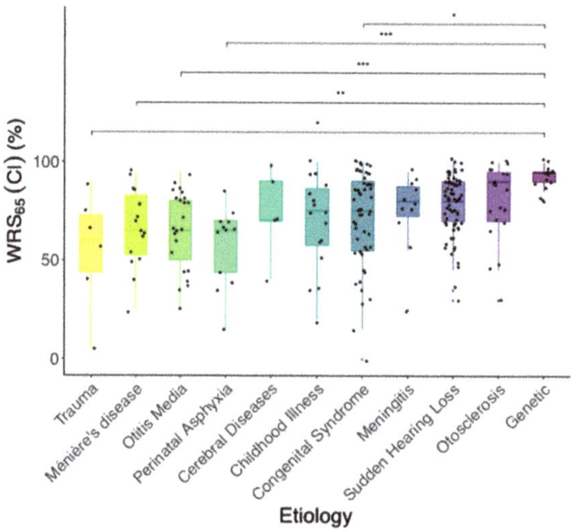

Figure 5. Box-whisker plots of WRS_{65}(CI) for different etiologies of hearing loss. The order of the plots is based on the ascending median values from left to right. The density and dispersion of the data points demonstrate the frequency of each etiology and the distribution of postoperative outcomes. Data points represent individual ears. * represents $p < 0.05$, ** represents $p < 0.01$ and *** represents $p < 0.001$.

(2) In the Kruskal–Wallis-Test, a statistically significant effect of the etiology of hearing loss on WRS_{65}(CI) ($\chi^2 = 36.75$, $p < 0.05$) was found. Five out of the 55 pairwise comparisons of the etiologies (corrected with Holm) showed a significant difference in WRS_{65}(CI). On the group median, cases with the etiology "Congenital", "Trauma", "Meniere's disease", "Otitis media" or "Perinatal asphyxia" revealed worse postoperative speech understanding compared to genetic hearing loss.

3.4. Validation of the Prediction Model

Figure 6 shows the frequency distribution of the prediction error calculated as the difference between the actual word recognition with CI after at least 6 months and the predicted word recognition according to Equation (1). In all cases with a positive difference, the predicted word recognition was exceeded, whereas all cases with a negative difference did not achieve the prediction. In the present population of 601 cases with a mWRS > 0%, the prediction was missed by more than 20 percentage points (pp) downward in 77 cases (12.8%).

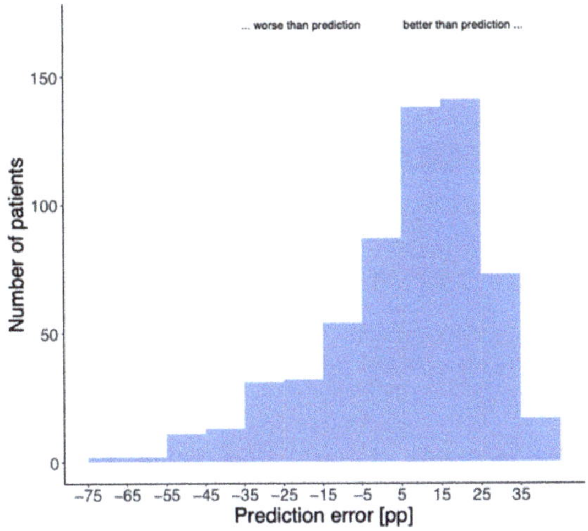

Figure 6. Frequency distribution of the differences between measured and predicted WRS_{65}(CI) based on Equation (1). In all cases with negative values, the prediction was not achieved.

The median absolute error of the prediction according to Equation (1) is 16.1 pp. Table 3 summarizes the effect of the etiology on selected location parameters of the distribution with respect to the results of the total population (left columns "Absolute" and "Relative to Model"; the latter have been corrected by the above-mentioned 9.9 pp to improve the visualization of the lower dispersion attributable to etiologies). Cases with genetic hearing loss exhibited significantly better WRS_{65}(CI) than the whole population. In contrast, cases with perinatal asphyxia showed significantly below-average WRS_{65}(CI). Regarding model error, only cases with perinatal asphyxia were found to have significantly worse than predicted WRS_{65}(CI). Overall, consideration of etiology with respect to the model leads to a significantly lower deviation from the prediction for the total population (sign test: $p = 5 \times 10^{-4}$, expressed by the model error). From the difference in p-values for WRS_{65}(CI) and model error, it follows that preoperative mWRS and WRS_{65}(HA) partly include the effect of etiology on WRS_{65}(CI).

Table 3. Effect of etiology on word recognition with CI at 65 dB SPL on the model error and its interquartile range.

	Absolute			Relative to Model			
Etiology	**Number of Cases**	**Mean WRS_{65}(CI)**	**Difference to Median WRS_{65}(CI)**	**Median Error [pp]**	**Adjusted Median Error [pp]**	**Interquartile Range of Error**	**Number of Cases Where Prediction Is Missed by More than 20 pp**
Genetic hearing loss	14	95	15	15. 5	5.5	17.3	0 (0%)
Sudden hearing loss	66	80	0	11.0	1.0	21.2	3 (5%)
Childhood illness	16	75	−5	10.8	0.9	26.5	3 (20%)
Congenital syndrome	54	75	−5	9.5	−0.5	31.9	10 (19%)
Meningitis	11	80	0	15.0	5.1	14.6	2 (18%)
Ménière's disease	15	65	−15	−1.8	−11.7	33.7	2 (13%)
Otitis media	23	65	−15	2.2	−7.7	35.7	5 (22%)
Otosclerosis	21	90	10	16.3	6.3	22.7	1 (5%)
Perinatal asphyxia	12	65	−15	−6.8	−16.8	29.7	4 (33%)
Trauma	6	60	−20	−6.2	−16.1	34.0	1 (17%)
Unknown	358	80	0	10.7	0.8	23.1	45 (13%)
Cerebral diseases	5	70	−10	6.2	−3.7	35.8	1 (20%)
Total	601	80	0	9.9	0	17.3	77 (13%)

For some etiologies (perinatal asphyxia, Menière's disease, genetic hearing loss, otitis media, trauma, and cerebral disease), interquartile ranges of model error greater than 30 pp can be identified. These are not equivalent to a worse prediction on average but indicate much greater variability that cannot be explained by the model within the corresponding patient groups.

4. Discussion

Of the 494 cases with available data on word recognition with HA at 65 dB SPL, 472 (95.5%) had significantly better speech understanding with CI at at least six months compared with preoperative HA, and one case showed a significantly poorer outcome. Overall word recognition improved by 64 pp to 74%.

The clinical relevance of maximum monosyllabic word recognition as a minimum outcome predictor was confirmed within this retrospective study in the largest patient population to date using the inclusion criterion of a preoperative mWRS greater than zero percent. In only 3% of the cases, the mWRS could not be achieved with CI.

The model for estimating the postoperative WRS_{65}(CI) according to Equation (1) were confirmed by the data of our patients. The median absolute error of the prediction according to Equation (1) is 16.1 pp. This is a higher deviation than the 11 or 14 pp reported by Hoppe et al. [17,19]. However, the median error of 9.9 pp found in our study reveals that this higher absolute error can be justified by the overall result above prediction and, thus, by an even better result than predicted. The model according to Equation (1) refers to six-monthly values for the WRS_{65}(CI), whereas six-month and later time points were analyzed in the present retrospective study.

As previously described in a very large patient collective with 2251 patients [15], etiology had a significant effect on postoperative speech understanding in the present study. For the subpopulation with a genetic cause of hearing loss, both studies found a relatively small but significant positive effect on WRS_{65}(CI). In contrast, Blamey et al. [15] determined above-average results for Menière's disease, whereas we report a median WRS_{65}(CI) of 15 pp below the value for the total population for the included 15 cases. This might be attributable to one inclusion criterion. Whereas Blamey et al. probably included mainly cases without preoperative speech understanding, i.e., presumably with inactive Menière's disease, we only included cases with mWRS greater than zero, i.e., Menière's disease was still active. This particular cohort of patients presents a challenge in the context of postoperative rehabilitation and programming because of persistent distortions in auditory perception [21]. Fluctuations in speech understanding with CI are to be expected in patients with persistent auditory fluctuations because of active disease. Although long-term care outcomes for inactive Menière's disease have been described as good [21], active Menière's still requires considerable clinical or individual resources [22,23]. The impact on WRS_{65}(CI) and subjective hearing-related impairment might be substantial [21,22,24]. Previous studies have demonstrated that patients with active Menière's and fluctuating hearing have increased impedances and require continuous adjustments to the CI sound processor [25]. Kanona et al. [21], suggest that patients with Menière's disease are likely to require a longer rehabilitation period after cochlear implantation.

4.1. Etiology and Modeling

Compared with the differences in WRS_{65}(CI) between the individual etiologies and the total population, the model errors for the results of the WRS_{65}(CI) for the various etiologies show significantly lower variability (see Table 3). This lower variability suggests that much of the variability, as described by Blamey et al. [15] for the different etiologies, are explained by the preoperatively collected data. In addition, we assume that, especially for the negative-impact etiologies, our patient population represents a positive selection. For example, the included cases of meningitis represent rather mild courses because, as per inclusion criteria, a preoperative mWRS greater than zero was still measurable, and thus no ossification of the cochlea or no or only limited degeneration of the spiral ganglion cells was present. As a rule, CI patients who become deaf following meningitis have worse long-term hearing and speech results [15,26].

We observed the largest negative deviations between measured and predicted WRS_{65}(CI), i.e., the largest negative model errors for the etiologies of Menière's disease, perinatal asphyxia, and trauma, which were accompanied by comparatively higher interquartile ranges of this error. The highest rate of cases missing the prognosis by more than 20 pp was detected in patients with perinatal asphyxia (33%). The lowest deviations in this respect are to be expected for cases with genetic hearing loss, hearing loss, and otosclerosis.

The few patients with a comparatively good 4PTA (<70 dB HL, $n = 43$) and conspicuously low speech understanding represent a constellation that is currently still insufficiently explained. The same applies to cases with very high mWRS, which cannot be approximately achieved with HA at 65 dB SPL. Although we and other clinics [13,14,17,19] can report successful cochlear implantation in this small group of patients, the reasons for this discrepancy between the preoperative unaided pure-tone average hearing threshold and speech understanding remain largely unknown and need to be clarified. There are indications that these cases are to be expected more frequently with increasing age [27]. The objective clarification of these cases appears difficult, as findings that can be clearly interpreted, e.g., via electrocochleography, seem to show a lower incidence with increasing age [28]. Deprivational processes within the auditory periphery offer a possible explanation [29]. Reduced top-down functions, such as impaired linguistic and neurocognitive abilities, should also be considered as a possible cause [30]. To the best of our knowledge, however, no established or scalable methods exist for assessing these functions in routine clinical practice. In summary, despite the currently limited understanding of the pathogenesis and differential diagnosis and the lack of alternative forms of therapy, cochlear implantation is, in the majority of cases, a successful therapy for improving the limited speech understanding obtained with HA preoperatively.

4.2. Limits of This Study

In this retrospective study, we were unable to assess the individual WRS_{65}(CI) at the six-month time point in all cases suggested by Hoppe et al. [17]. In addition, the COVID pandemic made the scheduled collection of postoperative speech understanding difficult [31]. A meta-analysis of the development of speech understanding showed rapid and significant improvement within the first three months after the first fitting, with no further statistically significant improvement after three months for the average patient [32]. Firszt et al. [16] have also stated that 90% of the final score can be expected after six to seven months. Thus, compared with Hoppe et al. [17], the various measurement times of our work do not bring into question the validity of the mWRS as a minimum predictor, the applicability of the prediction according to Equation (1), or the influence of etiology.

We were also unable to examine the influence of the rehabilitation process on postoperative speech understanding at our clinic, including the sound processor fitting, due to the retrospective study design. It can be assumed that in the case of known comorbidities, there will be greater deviations in the CI rehabilitation and consequently in the WRS_{65}(CI). A possible negative influence of comorbidities on postoperative speech understanding could thus be mitigated. A recent study [33] successfully applied the model [17] to systematically relate WRS_{65}(CI) deviations from prediction to postoperative audiometry results. By extending the model, the results of Dziemba et al. [33] may offer an explanation for the observed poorer WRS_{65}(CI) via significantly poorer audibility in the high-frequency range and possibly insufficient or incorrectly weighted loudness in the different frequency ranges.

Hoppe et al. [19] point out that the prediction via the model or individual deviations from it now influence the processes within postoperative rehabilitation at their clinics. This was not the case in the present retrospective study with cases that were partly treated 18 years ago. In this respect, the number of cases reported here, which miss the prognosis by more than 20 pp, is rather an upper estimate. This means that, fortunately, the prognosis is exceeded by the majority of patients, and only a small proportion of patients do not achieve the prognosis for postoperative speech understanding.

Even though bilateral hearing does play a role in the context of CI provision, this study treated ears separately according to the German CI guidelines and clinical practice [1,5,12–14,17,19,34]. To our knowledge, there is no validated model for predicting WRS that can be populated with our baseline audiometric data from the CI ears of both unilateral and bilateral implanted patients. There is a certain but yet unknown variability due to the neglection of contralateral hearing. Within this retrospective study, the corresponding data are not available to a sufficient degree. Further studies are needed to investigate the impact of contralateral hearing loss with respect to outcome prediction.

Further pre- and postoperative studies, including a larger number of patients with rare etiologies and the inclusion of early intervention based on the clear formulation of therapeutic goals for the WRS_{65}(CI), therefore seem very reasonable.

5. Conclusions

Cochlear implantation of patients with preoperatively measurable speech understanding with optimized HA having sufficient amplification power (HA classified as WHO 4) and a WRS with a HA below 60% represents a promising therapy option. This treatment should even be considered for patients with an average pure tone hearing loss of 60 dB HL (in some individual cases, even below this value) if the fitting of a HA is not successful.

We can confirm the use of preoperative maximum word recognition as a minimum predictor for the postoperative word recognition achievable with CI at 65 dB SPL in our extensive patient population. Moreover, this prediction can be further refined with the model used here. Part of the large interindividual variability in postoperative speech understanding attributable to various etiologies can be explained by the preoperative speech understanding included in the model. For some etiologies, greater variability in outcomes and deviations from prediction have been observed. These should be considered when counseling patients and planning postoperative rehabilitation.

Author Contributions: Conceptualization, S.A. and A.A.; methodology, S.A. and R.C.; software, R.C.; validation, S.A. and R.C.; formal analysis, S.A., R.C. and T.W.; investigation, S.A. and A.A.; resources, R.C.; data curation, R.C. and S.A.; writing—original draft preparation, R.C., T.H. and S.A.; writing—review and editing, R.C., S.A., T.W., T.H., A.A., R.L.B. and M.C.K.; visualization, R.C.; supervision, S.A.; project administration, S.A.; funding none. All authors have read and agreed to the published version of the manuscript.

Funding: This research received no external funding.

Institutional Review Board Statement: The study was conducted in accordance with the Declaration of Helsinki and approved by the Ethics Committee of the University of Freiburg (EK-Freiburg: 23-1029-S1-retro, 9 March 2023).

Informed Consent Statement: Patient consent was waived due to the following reasons: The planned study data originates from our own research, and it is expected to be highly time-consuming and likely unfeasible to obtain patient consent for data use in this specific study. This is because the data collection goes back quite some time, and some patients may have changed their contact information or may no longer be alive. The effort required to collect consent is disproportionate, and it is more practical to utilize the data after pseudonymization without obtaining individual consent. According to the balancing of interests outlined in § 13 Abs. 1 LDSG-BW, it can be assumed that the interest in conducting this study outweighs the interests of the individuals in excluding data processing. This can be justified by the fulfillment of criteria for scientific research, adherence to data processing requirements, and the assurance of guarantees described in the principles of personal data usage.

Data Availability Statement: Research data are available on request from the last author.

Conflicts of Interest: S. Arndt discloses the following: Advanced Bionics: travel reimbursement, financial support for research; Cochlear: financial support for research, travel reimbursement; MED-EL: financial support for research, travel reimbursement; Oticon Medical: travel reimbursement, financial support for research. T. Wesarg states the following: Advanced Bionics: financial support for research, travel reimbursement; Cochlear: financial support for research, travel reimbursement; MED-EL: financial support for research, travel reimbursement. A. Aschendorff states the following: Advanced Bionics: financial support for research, medical advisory board, travel reimbursement; Cochlear: financial support for research, travel reimbursement; MED-EL: financial support for research, travel reimbursement; Oticon Medical: financial support for research, travel reimbursement. Sensorion: financial support for research. M. C. Ketterer discloses the following: Cochlear: financial support for research, travel reimbursement; Oticon Medical: travel reimbursement, financial support for research; Sensorion: financial support for research. R. L. Beck discloses the following: Cochlear: financial support for research, travel reimbursement; Sensorion: financial support for research. T.H. is working for Cochlear Deutschland GmbH and Co., KG.

References

1. National Institute for Health and Care Excellence. Cochlear Implants for Children and Adults with Severe to Profound Deafness. 2019. Available online: https://www.nice.org.uk/guidance/ta566 (accessed on 23 October 2023).
2. AWMF. Leitlinien: Cochlea-Implantat Versorgung und Zentral-Auditorische Implantate. 2020. Available online: https://www.awmf.org/uploads/tx_szleitlinien/017-071l_S2k_Cochlea-Implantat-Versorgung-zentral-auditorische-Implantate_2020-12.pdf (accessed on 23 October 2023).
3. Van der Straaten, T.F.K.; Briaire, J.J.; Vickers, D.; Boermans, P.; Frijns, J.H.M. Selection Criteria for Cochlear Implantation in the United Kingdom and Flanders: Toward a Less Restrictive Standard. *Ear Hear.* **2020**, *42*, 68. [CrossRef] [PubMed]
4. Buchman, C.A.; Gifford, R.H.; Haynes, D.S.; Lenarz, T.; O'Donoghue, G.; Adunka, O.; Biever, A.; Briggs, R.J.; Carlson, M.L.; Dai, P.; et al. Unilateral Cochlear Implants for Severe, Profound, or Moderate Sloping to Profound Bilateral Sensorineural Hearing Loss: A Systematic Review and Consensus Statements. *JAMA Otolaryngol.-Head Neck Surg.* **2020**, *146*, 942–953. [CrossRef] [PubMed]
5. DGHNO-KHC. Weißbuch Cochlea-Implantat(CI)-Versorgung, 2nd Edition. 2021. Available online: https://cdn.hno.org/media/2021/ci-weissbuch-20-inkl-anlagen-datenblocke-und-zeitpunkte-datenerhebung-mit-logo-05-05-21.pdf (accessed on 23 October 2023).
6. Gifford, R.H.; Dorman, M.F.; Shallop, J.K.; Sydlowski, S.A. Evidence for the expansion of adult cochlear implant candidacy. *Ear Hear.* **2010**, *31*, 186–194. [CrossRef] [PubMed]
7. Rauch, A.K.; Metzner, T.; Aschendorff, A.; Arndt, S.; Speck, I.; Laszig, R.; Beck, R.L. Speech processor upgrade increases speech comprehension in patients with cochlear implants. *HNO* **2019**, *67*, 778–785. [CrossRef] [PubMed]
8. Wesarg, T.; Voss, B.; Hassepass, F.; Beck, R.; Aschendorff, A.; Laszig, R.; Arndt, S. Speech Perception in Quiet and Noise With an Off the Ear CI Processor Enabling Adaptive Microphone Directionality. *Otol. Neurotol.* **2018**, *39*, e240–e249. [CrossRef] [PubMed]
9. Aschendorff, A.; Briggs, R.; Brademann, G.; Helbig, S.; Hornung, J.; Lenarz, T.; Marx, M.; Ramos, A.; Stöver, T.; Escudé, B.; et al. Clinical investigation of the Nucleus Slim Modiolar Electrode. *Audiol. Neurotol.* **2017**, *22*, 169–179. [CrossRef]
10. Aschendorff, A.; Klenzner, T.; Arndt, S.; Beck, R.; Schild, C.; Röddiger, L.; Maier, W.; Laszig, R. Insertion results for Contour and Contour Advance electrodes: Are there individual learning curves? *HNO* **2011**, *59*, 448–452. [CrossRef]
11. Hey, M.; Böhnke, B.; Mewes, A.; Munder, P.; Mauger, S.J.; Hocke, T. Speech comprehension across multiple CI processor generations: Scene dependent signal processing. *Laryngoscope Investig. Otolaryngol.* **2021**, *6*, 807–815. [CrossRef]

12. Hoppe, U.; Hocke, T.; Hast AIro, H. Maximum preimplantation monosyllabic score as predictor of cochlear implant outcome. *HNO* **2019**, *67*, 62–68. [CrossRef]
13. Thangavelu, K.; Nitzge, M.; Weiß, R.M.; Mueller-Mazzotta, J.; Stuck, B.A.; Reimann, K. Role of cochlear reserve in adults with cochlear implants following post-lingual hearing loss. *Eur. Arch. Oto-Rhino-Laryngol.* **2022**, *280*, 1063–1071. [CrossRef]
14. Rieck, J.H.; Beyer, A.; Mewes, A.; Caliebe, A.; Hey, M. Extended Preoperative Audiometry for Outcome Prediction and Risk Analysis in Patients Receiving Cochlear Implants. *J. Clin. Med.* **2023**, *12*, 3262. [CrossRef] [PubMed]
15. Blamey, P.; Artieres, F.; Başkent, D.; Bergeron, F.; Beynon, A.; Burke, E.; Dillier, N.; Dowell, R.; Fraysse, B.; Gallégo, S.; et al. Factors affecting auditory performance of postlinguistically deaf adults using cochlear implants: An update with 2251 patients. *Audiol. Neuro-Otol.* **2013**, *18*, 36–47. [CrossRef] [PubMed]
16. Holden, L.K.; Finley, C.C.; Firszt, J.B.; Holden, T.A.; Brenner, C.; Potts, L.G.; Gotter, B.D.; Vanderhoof, S.S.; Mispagel, K.; Heydebrand, G.; et al. Factors affecting open-set word recognition in adults with cochlear implants. *Ear Hear.* **2013**, *34*, 342–360. [CrossRef] [PubMed]
17. Hoppe, U.; Hocke, T.; Hast, A.; Iro, H. Cochlear Implantation in Candidates With Moderate-to-Severe Hearing Loss and Poor Speech Perception. *Laryngoscope* **2021**, *131*, E940–E945. [CrossRef] [PubMed]
18. Shafieibavani, E.; Goudey, B.; Kiral, I.; Zhong, P.; Jimeno-Yepes, A.; Swan, A.; Gambhir, M.; Buechner, A.; Kludt, E.; Eikelboom, R.H.; et al. Predictive models for cochlear implant outcomes: Performance, generalizability, and the impact of cohort size. *Trends Hear.* **2021**, *25*, 23312165211066174. [CrossRef] [PubMed]
19. Hoppe, U.; Hast, A.; Hocke, T. Validation of a predictive model for speech discrimination after cochlear implant provision. *HNO* **2023**, *71*, 53–59. [CrossRef] [PubMed]
20. Winkler, A.; Holube, I. Test-retest reliability of the Freiburg monosyllabic speech test. *HNO* **2016**, *64*, 564–571. [CrossRef] [PubMed]
21. Kanona, H.; Forde, C.; Van Rooyen, A.M.; Keating, P.; Bradley, J.; Pendolino, A.L.; Mehta, N.; Manjaly, J.G.; Khalil, S.; Lavy, J.; et al. Cochlear implant outcomes in patients with Meniere's disease: A large case series. *Cochlear Implant. Int.* **2022**, *23*, 339–346. [CrossRef]
22. Hast, A.; Meßbacher, M.E.; Liebscher, T.; Hornung, J.; Hoppe, U. Fluctuation in electrical hearing in a Morbus Meniere's patient. *Clin. Case Rep.* **2021**, *9*, e04411. [CrossRef]
23. Pfeiffer, C.J.; Gehl, H.B.; Scholtz, L.U.; Goon, P.; Sudhoff, H.; Todt, I. Endolymphatic Hydrops Magnet Resonance Imaging in Ménière's Disease Patients after Cochlea Implantation. *Brain Sci.* **2023**, *13*, 853. [CrossRef]
24. Wrobel, C.; Bevis, N.F.; Klinge-Strahl, A.; Strenzke, N.; Beutner, D. Performance and self-perceived hearing impairment after cochlear implantation in Menière's disease. *Laryngoscope Investig. Otolaryngol.* **2022**, *7*, 219–225. [CrossRef] [PubMed]
25. Samy, R.N.; Houston, L.; Scott, M.; Choo, D.I.; Meinzen-Derr, J. Cochlear implantation in patients with Meniere's disease. *Cochlear Implant. Int.* **2016**, *16*, 208–212. [CrossRef] [PubMed]
26. Altuntaş, O.M.; Özkan, B.; Bajin, D.; Sennaroğlu, G.; Sennaroğlu, L. Long-Term Outcome of Cochlear Implantation in Post-meningitic Deafness. *J. Int. Adv. Otol.* **2021**, *17*, 500–507. [CrossRef] [PubMed]
27. Hoppe, U.; Hocke, T.; Iro, H. Age-Related Decline of Speech Perception. *Front. Aging Neurosci.* **2022**, *14*, 891202. [CrossRef] [PubMed]
28. Riggs, W.J.; Roche, J.P.; Giardina, C.K.; Harris, M.S.; Bastian, Z.J.; Fontenot, T.E.; Buchman, C.A.; Brown, K.D.; Adunka, O.F.; Fitzpatrick, D.C. Intraoperative Electrocochleographic Characteristics of Auditory Neuropathy Spectrum Disorder in Cochlear Implant Subjects. *Front. Neurosci.* **2017**, *11*, 416. [CrossRef] [PubMed]
29. Walger, M.; Foerst, A.; Beutner, D.; Streicher, B.; Stürmer, K.; Lang-Roth, R. Auditory synaptopathy/neuropathy: Clinical findings and diagnosis. *HNO* **2011**, *59*, 414–424. [CrossRef]
30. Moberly, A.C.; Bates, C.; Harris, M.S.; Pisoni, D.B. The Enigma of Poor Performance by Adults With Cochlear Implants. *Otol. Neurotol.* **406**, 2014; 1522-1528. [CrossRef]
31. Aschendorff, A.; Arndt, S.; Kröger, S.; Wesarg, T.; Ketterer, M.C.; Kirchem, P.; Pixner, S.; Hassepaß, F.; Beck, R. Quality of cochlear implant rehabilitation under COVID-19 conditions. *HNO* **2021**, *69*, 1–6. [CrossRef]
32. Ma, C.; Fried, J.; Nguyen, S.A.; Schvartz-Leyzac, K.C.; Camposeo, E.L.; Meyer, T.A.; Dubno, J.R.; McRackan, T.R. Longitudinal Speech Recognition Changes After Cochlear Implant: Systematic Review and Meta-analysis. *Laryngoscope* **2023**, *133*, 1014–1024. [CrossRef]
33. Dziemba, O.C.; Merz, S.; Hocke, T. Evaluative audiometry after cochlear implant provision. German Version. *HNO* **2023**, *72*, 56–62. [CrossRef]
34. Patro, A.; Lindquist, N.R.; Holder, J.T.; Tawfik, K.O.; O'Malley, M.R.; Bennett, M.L.; Haynes, D.S.; Gifford, R.; Perkins, E.L. Further Evidence for Individual Ear Consideration in Cochlear Implant Candidacy Evaluation. *Otol. Neurotol.* **2022**, *43*, 1033–1040. [CrossRef] [PubMed]

Journal of
Clinical Medicine

MDPI

Article

Word Recognition with a Cochlear Implant in Relation to Prediction and Electrode Position

Annett Franke-Trieger *, Susen Lailach, Joshua Shetty, Katrin Murrmann, Thomas Zahnert and Marcus Neudert

Department of Otorhinolaryngology, Head and Neck Surgery, Faculty of Medicine Carl Gustav Carus, Technische Universität Dresden, Fetscherstraße 74, 01307 Dresden, Germany; thomas.zahnert@ukdd.de (T.Z.)
* Correspondence: annett.trieger@ukdd.de

Abstract: Background: the word recognition score (WRS) achieved with cochlear implants (CIs) varies widely. To account for this, a predictive model was developed based on patients' age and their pre-operative WRS. This retrospective study aimed to find out whether the insertion depth of the nucleus lateral-wall electrode arrays contributes to the deviation of the CI-achieved WRS from the predicted WRS. Materials and methods: patients with a pre-operative maximum WRS > 0 or a pure-tone audiogram ≥80 dB were included. The insertion depth was determined via digital volume tomography. Results: fifty-three patients met the inclusion criteria. The median WRS achieved with the CI was 70%. The comparison of pre- and post-operative scores achieved with a hearing aid and a CI respectively in the aided condition showed a median improvement of 65 percentage points (pp). A total of 90% of the patients improved by at least 20 pp. The majority of patients reached or exceeded the prediction, with a median absolute error of 11 pp. No significant correlation was found between the deviation from the predicted WRS and the insertion depth. Conclusions: our data support a previously published model for the prediction of the WRS after cochlear implantation. For the lateral-wall electrode arrays evaluated, the insertion depth did not influence the WRS with a CI.

Keywords: cochlear implant; WRS prediction; insertion depth; word recognition score; lateral wall; digital volume tomography

1. Introduction

Cochlear implantation is an established treatment option for patients with hearing loss for which hearing aids (HAs) or other less invasive options have failed to restore speech perception to a sufficient degree [1]. The vast majority of cochlear implant (CI) recipients show improved word recognition scores (WRSs) if the pre-operative-aided scores at a conversational level of 65 dB (WRS_{65}(HA)) and post-operative scores with a CI (WRS_{65}(CI)) are compared [2–9]. A number of pre-, intra- and post-operatively assessed outcome-predicting factors have been identified [2–7]. Blamey et al. found five intrinsic factors that had an impact on the post-operative word recognition score: the duration and age of onset of severe-to-profound hearing loss, age at the time of surgery, aetiology, and implant experience. Additionally, Holden et al. [3] identified extrinsic factors, such as scalar location, insertion depth, array insertion depth, angular position of the basal electrode's contact, and wrapping factor as affecting word recognition.

Recent studies [10–12] have revealed the variability in electrode array positioning. This is partially due to differences in cochlear size, scalar shifts, and different electrode designs [13–15]), causing different electrophysiological findings [16] and different intra-cochlear trajectories of the electrode array [17]. In measurements in vivo, the insertion depth angle (AID) was found to vary by up to 300° for certain electrode arrays [10].

Placement shift due to scalar shift did not result in coherent findings with respect to speech comprehension. Liebscher et al. [12] did not find measurable differences in the WRS, whereas Aschendorff et al. [18] reported a detrimental effect of dislocation of up to

10 percentage points (pp) for the WRS of patients with scalar dislocations. Furthermore, the surgeon represents another source of variability in the electrode's position; this might be intended for certain techniques, such as the pull-back technique [19,20], or be due to the placement of the electrode array in the markings specified by the implant manufacturers, which can cause variability in the distance between the first electrode's contact and the round window, depending on the electrode array.

The position of the electrode array does affect electrophysiological measures, such as electrically evoked compound action potential, ECAP [11]. Therefore, the question arises of whether the electrode position has an influence on a CI's performance.

However, for the comparison of both perimodiolar and lateral-wall electrode arrays and the influence of insertion depth, no consistent results have been shown; this may be due in part to the inhomogeneity of the patient groups analysed.

To account for the variability in audiological outcomes, significant efforts in recent years have focused on developing valid and reliable predictive models. In recent studies, Hoppe et al. proposed [5] and validated [9] a prediction model with a comparatively low prediction error (mean absolute error, MAE) of 11.5 pp [7,9].

$$WRS_{65}(CI)[\%] = \frac{100}{1 + e^{-(\beta_0 + \beta_1 \cdot WRS_{max} + \beta_2 \cdot age + \beta_3 \cdot WRS_{65}(HA))}} \tag{1}$$

with $\beta_0 = 0.84 \pm 0.18$ $\beta_1 = 0.012 \pm 0.0015\ 1/\%$ $\beta_2 = -0.0094 \pm 0.0025\ 1/\text{years}$ $\beta_3 = 0.0059 \pm 0.0026\ 1/\%$.

The model is based on pre-operative audiometric measures only: the maximum word recognition score (WRS_{max}), the WRS_{65}(HA), and the recipient's age at implantation. This outcome prediction model can facilitate the pre-operative counselling of HA users [5,21]. Furthermore, Hoppe et al. found that the WRS_{max} is a highly reliable minimum predictor [4]. Both of these measures can be used within post-operative CI aftercare to set an expectation value (and post-operative objective) for WRS_{65}(CI). This predicted WRS_{65}(CI) can be used to monitor and reference the patient's progress and, if appropriate, to reallocate clinical resources to improve outcomes [9]. In a recent study [22], the model was applied to investigate the systematic differences between CI recipients' reaching or missing the predicted WRS_{65}(CI). For this purpose, Dziemba et al. [22] expanded the exponential term in Equation (1) with additional factors representing post-operative audibility and loudness growths. They found that there are systematic differences between poor- and well-performing subjects; these differences are basically due to CI system fitting.

To our knowledge, this model has not yet been used to investigate contributing factors such as electrode positioning [3].

In the evaluation of the electrode array position, a distinction must be clear between lateral-wall and perimodiolar electrode arrays. While Liebscher et al. [12] determined the relationships between surgical technique, speech perception, electrophysiological parameters, and scalar translocations for perimodiolar electrode arrays, no information exists yet on the influence of surgical insertion on outcomes when a lateral-wall electrode of the same implant generation is used. On one hand, prediction models can contribute to more precise patient counselling, and on the other, they can be used for quality assurance measures, since a precise therapy target can be defined. In cases of deviation from the prognosis, pre-operative parameters (anamnesis, aetiology, and anatomy), intra-operative factors (electrode array insertion), and post-operative aspects (fitting and rehabilitation strategy) have to be examined.

Consequently, this study aimed to answer the question of whether optimising intra-operative process quality (i.e., in this case, by optimising the insertion depth) can reduce the deviation from the predicted WRS. Furthermore, one must ask whether the insertion depth contributes to the variability in the deviation from the prediction. The relationship between angular insertion depth and cochlear size, as well as the influence of the surgeon, was investigated. By varying the insertion depth alone, the surgeon could potentially contribute to the variability in the outcome of cochlear implantation.

In this study, we analysed the WRS to determine the influence of electrode position (the angular insertion depth and the distance between the most basal electrode contact and the round window).

2. Materials and Methods

2.1. Subjects

We reviewed all adult patients who received a Cochlear™ Nucleus® implant (Cochlear Ltd., Sydney, Australia) with lateral-wall electrode arrays (CI522 or CI622) at the University Hospital of Dresden between May 2015 and June 2021. The two implant types have identical lateral-wall electrode arrays and functions. The receiver/stimulator housings differ. The inclusion criteria for this study were: sensorineural origin of hearing loss, post-lingual onset of deafness, native German speaker, imaging of the cochlea without pathological findings or malformations, age at implantation ≥18 years, and regular visits to the rehabilitation centre for fitting, audiometric testing, and hearing therapy. The hearing loss for air conduction was determined as the mean value over the frequencies 0.5, 1, 2, and 4 kHz (PTA4). For hearing thresholds beyond the maximum possible presentation levels of the audiometers, a value of 120 dB_{HL} was assigned. With respect to pure tone and speech audiometry, only patients with $WRS_{max} > 0\%$ or PTA4 ≥ 80 dB_{HL} were included. Furthermore, only patients with correct intracochlear electrode positioning were included. This was verified using a digital volume tomography image.

This study was conducted in accordance with the Declaration of Helsinki (2013) on research involving human subjects and was approved by the local ethics committee (SR+BO-260052021). The study was also registered under DRKS00026741 with the German register of clinical studies.

2.2. Audiometric Measures

Speech audiometry was performed using the Freiburg monosyllabic word test. The pre-operative WRS was measured with headphones in the unaided condition. To identify WRS_{max}, the presentation level was increased in steps of 10 dB until the maximum score achievable (WRS_{max}) below the patient's loudness discomfort level was reached [5]. The WRS in the aided condition, i.e., with hearing aids (WRS_{65}(HA)) and with the cochlear implant (WRS_{65}(CI)) was measured in an anechoic soundproof booth at a loudspeaker presentation level of 65 dB SPL, with the patient seated 1.0 m in front of the loudspeaker. The measurements were performed monaurally. If necessary, the contralateral ear was appropriately masked with wideband noise presented through the headphones (DT48; beyerdynamic GmbH & Co. KG, Heilbronn, Germany). Speech audiometry was performed with an AT900 or AT1000 clinical audiometer (Auritec GmbH, Hamburg, Germany). The WRS with the cochlear implant referred to the score measured twelve months after the first activation of the CI system. To calculate the prognoses of the WRS_{65}(CI), Equation (1) was used. Significant differences between WRSs were determined according to their critical differences according to Winkler and Holube [23].

2.3. Imaging

The flat panel volume tomography (digital volume tomography, DVT) examinations were carried out on the first day after implantation using a Flat Panel Computer Tomograph 3D Accuitomo 80 (J. Morita MFG. CORP., Kyoto, Japan). The imaging was performed with a tube current of 8 mA and a tube voltage of 90 kV. The raw projection images were reconstructed using i-dixl software (version 2.8., J. Morita MFG. CORP. Kyoto, Japan), resulting in a voxel size of 125 μm.

2.4. Measurement of Cochlear Diameter and Electrode Position

The angle and length measurements were performed according to the consensus paper [24] using the cochlear view, which is defined as the plane through the basal turn and perpendicular to the modiolus. Figure 1 shows an example of this measurement. The zero-degree reference angle was chosen at the centre of the round window according to the consensus paper. To quantify the cochlear size, the diameter of the basal turn of the cochlear was measured. This diameter is illustrated with the line that starts at the centre of the round window and crosses the position of the helicotrema and the ends of the lateral wall on the opposite side, as shown in earlier studies [25]. The distance, d, between the round window and the most basal electrode contact, was measured as shown in Figure 2. d is a parameter that describes how deeply the surgeon inserted the electrode array into the cochlea.

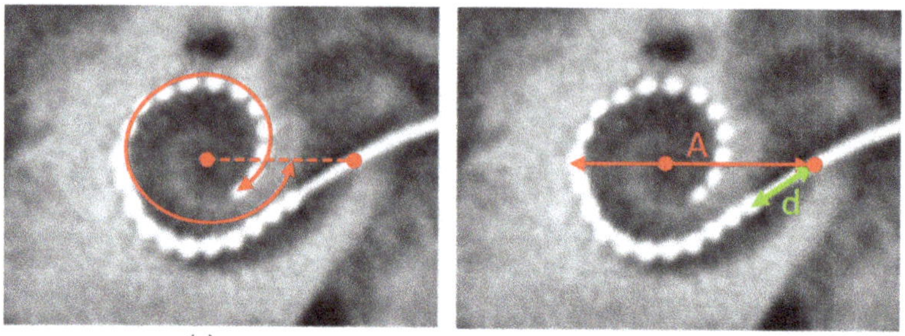

(a) (b)

Figure 1. Cochlear view of the DVT image with the red dots indicating the position of the modiolus and the position of the round window. (**a**) Measurement of the insertion depth angle. (**b**) Measurement of the diameter of the cochlear basal turn (A) and the distance between the round window and the most basal electrode contact (d).

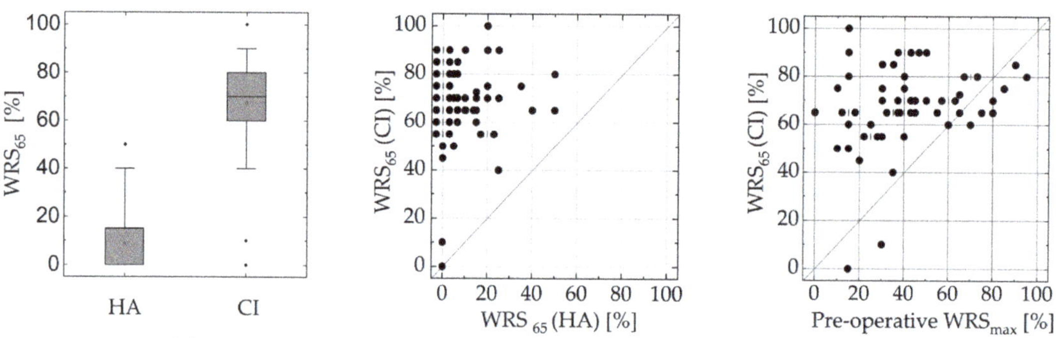

(a) (b) (c)

Figure 2. Relationship between pre- and post-operative audiometric measures. (**a**) Box plot comparing the pre-operative WRS_{65}(HA) and post-operative WRS_{65}(CI); the boxes show the quartiles and the whiskers show the 5th and 95th percentile; the median for HA lies on the lower edge of the box. (**b**) Scatter plot showing the same comparison. (**c**) Comparison between the pre-operative WRS_{max} and post-operative WRS_{65}(CI). In (**b**,**c**), the overlapping points are shifted apart horizontally, with a small vertical line representing their actual position.

2.5. Data Analysis

All analyses and figure creations were produced using OriginLab (version 2019, OriginLab software, Northampton, MA, USA). The correlation analysis was performed using Spearman's rank correlation method.

3. Results

3.1. Study Cases

Of 312 cochlear implantations carried out in the study period, 53 cases (i.e., individual ears; 34 right, 19 left) were identified that met the inclusion criteria. In all cases, implantation was carried out via round window insertion or via the extended round window approach. The implanted device was the CI522 in 37 cases and the CI622 in 16 cases. The age of the patients at implantation ranged from 26 to 80 years (mean: 61.4 years). The mean hearing loss for air conduction using the PTA4 was 80 $\pm$ 15 dB_{HL}.

Figure 2 shows the relationship between the pre- and post-operative WRSs. The median score achieved with the CI was 70% with the first quartile at 60% and the third quartile at 80%, as shown in Figure 2. Comparing the pre- and post-operative scores achieved in the aided condition showed a median improvement of 65 pp. In all cases, 90% improved by at least 20 pp. With respect to the minimum prediction, 96% of the recipients reached or exceeded the WRS_{max} while 83% of the recipients significantly exceeded the pre-operative WRS_{65}(HA) [23].

Figure 3 shows the distribution of differences between the measured and predicted WRSs (measured minus predicted). The differences range from −57 pp to +35 pp. The MAE was 11 pp. Three patients missed the predicted score by more than 20 pp.

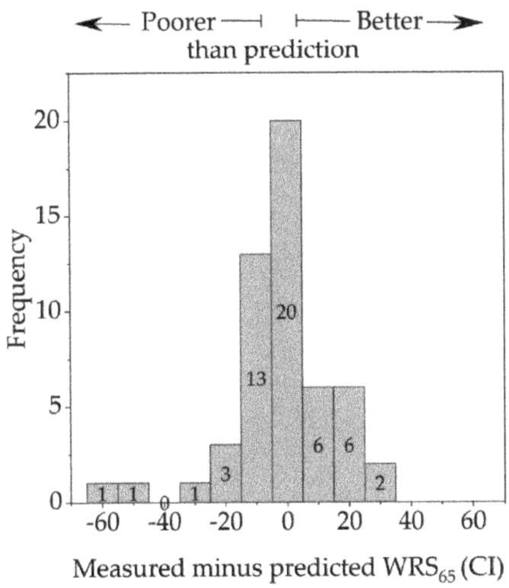

Figure 3. Distribution of differences (in percentage points) between the measured and predicted word recognition scores. Negative differences correspond to cases in which the measured scores were below the predictions.

3.2. Insertion Depth and Cochlear Size

Figure 4 shows the angular insertion depth as a function of the diameter (*A*) and of the distance, *d*, as defined in Figure 1. The diameter ranged from 8.05 mm to 10.34 mm. The median diameter was 8.96 mm. The distances, *d*, ranged from 1.5 mm to 8.3 mm. The median distance was 4.7 mm. The angular insertion depth ranged from 365° to 568°. The median angle was 460°.

A positive correlation was found between the distance, *d*, and the resulting angular insertion depth. A negative correlation was found between the cochlear diameter and angular insertion depth. The data show that the correlation between *d* and the angular insertion depth was stronger ($r = 0.673$, $p < 0.0001$) than the weak correlation between the angular insertion depth and cochlear diameter ($r = 0.306$, $p = 0.0254$).

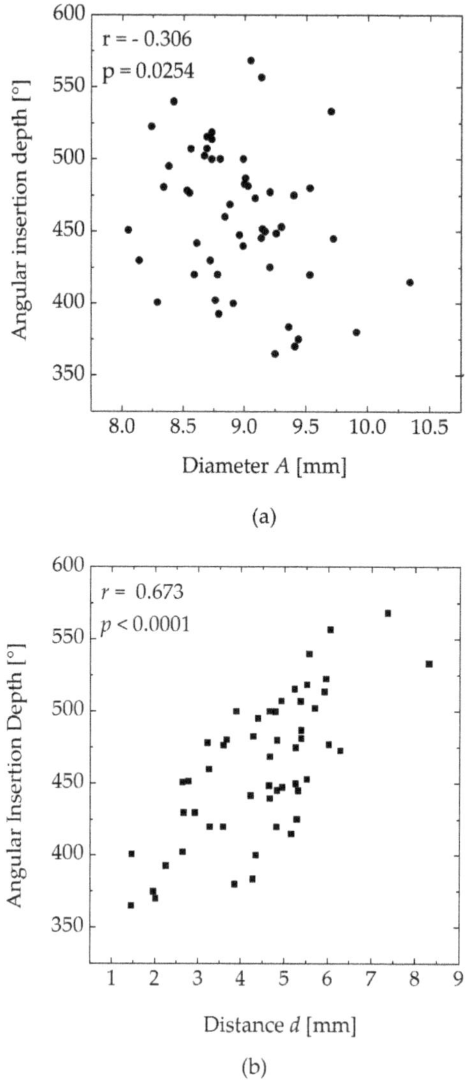

Figure 4. (**a**) Angular insertion depth as a function of the diameter of the basal turn A. (**b**) Angular insertion depth as a function of the distance, d, both defined in Figure 2. r, Spearman rank correlation coefficient.

3.3. Dependence of the WRS on the Electrode's Position and Cochlear Size

Figure 5 shows the difference between the measured and predicted WRSs as a function of the distance, d, and the angular insertion depth. The correlation analyses showed no significant correlation between the deviation from the predicted WRS and the distance d ($r = -0.256$, $p > 0.05$) and the angular insertion depth ($r = -0.185$, $p > 0.05$).

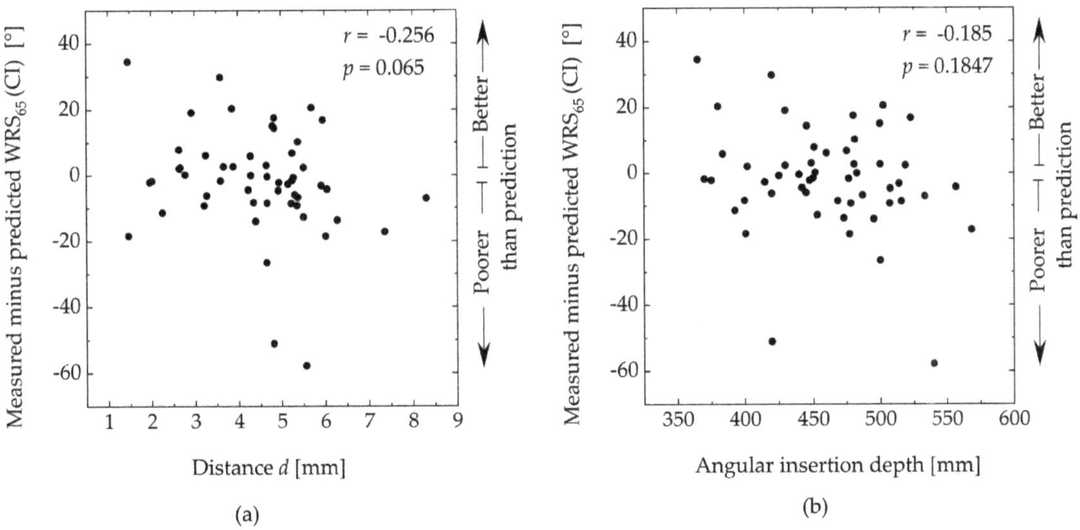

Figure 5. The difference between the measured and predicted word recognition scores as a function of (**a**) the distance, *d*, and (**b**) the angular insertion depth. *r*, Spearman rank correlation coefficient.

4. Discussion

The extension of the CI indication to patients who still have a capacity for speech perception inevitably creates enormous demands on the quality of care. In addition to pre-operative selection and counselling based on current audiological performance with and without a hearing aid, knowledge of potential surgical influencing factors and electrode array characteristics potentially contribute to the best possible hearing result by modulating these factors as necessary.

This study showed that 83% (44/53) of patients had clinically significantly ([23]; see also Methods) better WRSs after cochlear implantation than before with conventional hearing aids. The median improvement was 65 pp, and 90% of the patients showed an improvement of at least 20 pp. This is consistent with the results of earlier studies that also analysed word recognition with CIs in patients with residual hearing [4,8,26]. WRS_{65}(HA) alone is not suitable for predicting WRS_{65}(CI) post-operatively. Regression models only explain up to 10 pp of the WRS_{65}(CI) [5]. More than half of our patients had a pre-operative WRS_{65}(HA) of 0% even though the WRS_{max} was larger than zero. This finding, i.e., that the WRS_{max} is not met by the WRS_{65}(HA), is in accordance with the results of previous studies [4,5,8]. However, even this patient group was able to achieve a mean WRS_{65}(CI) of 65%, with a range from 0% to 90%. The inclusion of additional pre-operative speech audiometry measures may help to improve outcome prediction in this subgroup of recipients [26]. In contrast to WRS_{65}(HA), a stronger association of WRS_{65}(CI) with the pre-operative WRS_{max} was shown. Other research groups have already been able to identify this correlation [4,8,26]. These results suggest that patients with a pre-operatively great difference between WRS_{65}(HA) and WRS_{max} (speech perception gap) benefit from cochlear implantation [27]. Especially in patients with severe hearing loss, sufficient hearing aid fitting often fails, owing to technical limitations (feedback), the lack of acceptance of high sound levels, and a low dynamic range [28]. In our study, the WRS_{65}(CI) was below the WRS_{max} in only two patients. With respect to the minimum prediction, 96% of the recipients reached or exceeded their WRS_{max}.

The majority of patients achieved or exceeded the WRS_{65}(CI) predicted according to Equation (1). Three patients missed the predicted score by more than 20 pp. The prediction model was thus also confirmed with our study. In the validation process of the prediction model, Hoppe et al. [9] determined an MAE of 11.5 pp in a patient group with a WRS_{max} above zero. Additionally, they reported that 14 out of 85 patients missed the predicted score by more than 20 pp. For all patients with WRS_{max} = 0%, they reported an MAE of 23 pp. In our study, in cases with $WRS_{max} > 0$ or PTA4 $\geq$ 80 dB HL, the MAE was 11 pp.

The modelling of prognosis prediction by Hoppe et al. was based on a group of patients fitted with a perimodiolar electrode array. Our investigations confirm that the model can also be applied to patients with lateral-wall electrode arrays. In the current literature, no significant difference in speech comprehension between perimodiolar and lateral-wall electrode arrays can be found, although the heterogeneous quality of the studies does not allow a conclusive evaluation [29,30]. Especially for perimodiolar electrode arrays, the optimisation of the electrode array position is aimed at improving surgical techniques, e.g., the pullback technique, to achieve the smallest possible distance between the electrode array and the modiolus [19,31]. The results of our study suggest that such procedures are probably not necessary for the CI522/CI 622 implants, as the electrode array position ultimately has no influence on the audiological outcome.

While the pre-operative WRS_{max} could be confirmed as a strong minimum predictor, the insertion depth had no influence on the post-operative WRS_{65}(CI) in our study. The cochlear coverage could be influenced by the cochlear duct length (CDL) and the insertion depth of the electrode array. For CI systems with different available electrode lengths, the coverage is of course influenced by the chosen electrode's length. For the CI622/CI522 implants, the cochlear coverage is determined basically only by the CDL and the distance, *d* (first electrode contact to the round window). Up to now, no information has become available on the extent to which *d*, which ultimately is determined by the surgeon, influences post-operative performance. According to the physician's guide [32] provided by the implant company, the white markers, which are positioned 20 mm and 25 mm away from the apical tip of the electrode array, are currently used as a guide for insertion depth, and a maximum insertion depth of 25 mm is assumed. Deeper insertion was not considered necessary by the implant company, although no study data were presented to support this recommendation.

For other electrode manufacturers, especially those with different electrode lengths in their portfolio, the exact pre-operative planning of the electrode array position based on the CDL and the residual hearing was discussed [33]; however, this does not seem to be necessary for the CI622/CI 522 implants with normal cochlear anatomies. The influence of insertion depth on word recognition after implantation is frequently discussed in the current literature. While some authors have demonstrated better word recognition with deeper insertion in lateral-wall electrode arrays [34–37], this effect has been disputed by other research groups [38–40]. Some studies even showed a worse speech audiometric outcome with deeper insertion [38,41]. In most of these studies, all lateral-wall electrode arrays of all the available manufacturers were combined, so that no implant-specific recommendations could be derived from them. Other studies focused exclusively on implants from other manufacturers so the results cannot be applied to Nucleus implants, especially to the CI522/CI622 implants used in this study. Last but not least, the level of evidence of the current studies on the influence of insertion depth on audiological performance is currently not satisfactory [42]. Often, there is a lack of adequate consideration of additional known confounding factors and an adequate control group. The practice of switching off the apical electrode contacts to simulate a shortened insertion depth must also be critically questioned [40] since it is known that the number of active electrode contacts also contributes to word recognition.

Various hypotheses exist to explain the possible influence of insertion depth on post-operative word recognition. On the one hand, a greater insertion depth is considered to afford a better coverage of the spiral ganglia in the low-frequency range and a more physiological frequency assignment [40,43]. However, other authors presume a greater trauma for cochlear structures with deeper insertion [44]. In the case of shorter electrode arrays, individual authors have found a poorer outcome with deeper insertion, since the basal region is not sufficiently covered, owing to the greater distance between the first electrode contact and the round window [3,41]. This could not be confirmed in our study for the investigated electrode array of the CI622/CI 522 implants with an active length of 19.1 mm. Here, however, we should point out that these results cannot simply be transferred to electrode arrays from other companies. It should finally be observed that the debate regarding the ideal length of an electrode array and its ideal cochlear coverage, which has been going on for years (partly for reasons of marketing strategy) cannot at present be resolved.

The distance, d, from the first electrode contact to the round window, is the aspect of the insertion depth of the electrode array that can be determined and controlled by the surgeon himself. In our study, d was found to vary from 1.5 mm to 8.5 mm. When evaluating the scatter of d and insertion depth, the measurement error of the angle and length measurement based on the post-operative DVT must also be taken into account. In the literature, interrater differences of −0.5 to 0.5 mm for length measurements and 12° to 30° for angle measurements can be found [45].

In addition to the insertion depth, the aspect of structural preservation through atraumatic electrode insertion is currently under discussion. Therefore, studies are currently being performed to evaluate the influence of insertion speed and insertion force on the outcome of cochlear implantation. The preservation of residual hearing is primarily evaluated as a correlation of structural preservation. In recent years, electrocochleography has been implemented as a system for monitoring residual hearing in individual clinics [46–50]. Structural preservation as a function of insertion depth or residual hearing preservation was not assessed in our study. In the literature, the influence of insertion depth on residual hearing preservation is currently a topic of controversy. While some authors see the advantages of a lesser insertion depth, which is associated with less severe intracochlear trauma [44], other research groups have been able to demonstrate satisfactory residual hearing retention even with deeper insertion [51–53]. To summarise, at the moment is not clear how the WRS is affected by the factors discussed above. More studies are needed on the effect of these different factors on the WRS. To mention one example, Dalbert et al. [54] demonstrated better long-term speech understanding in patients with residual hearing than in the group of patients without residual hearing for patients with electrical stimulation alone. However, the significant positive effect in the study group was not seen until 18 months after CI activation.

Owing to the great heterogeneity of these studies, it is not currently possible to conduct a high-quality meta-analytical review of the relationship between insertion depth and speech comprehension. In a systematic review published in 2021 including seven studies with results of speech comprehension after one year, the effect of insertion depth could not be reliably assessed [42]. Because of the improvement in word recognition within the rehabilitation process, an assessment after less than 12 months does not seem to be very meaningful; however, after 12 months, stable speech comprehension can be assumed [3]. Interestingly, Büchner et al. [55] observed that the initially positive effect of a longer electrode array length diminished over the course of rehabilitation. The authors attributed this to cortical plasticity, which can compensate for any possible frequency mismatch present [55].

One limitation of our study is the lack of a systematic analysis of the fitting. Some studies have already shown the strong effect of fitting quality on the outcome of cochlear implantation. Thus, currently, high variability in audiological outcomes due to a less-than-optimum fitting is possible [22,56,57]. However, standardised quality indicators for the evaluation of fitting quality must be developed and analysed in further studies with the help of a prediction model. For example, by basing the adjustment on the electrode-specific ECAP or a categorical loudness scale, it should be possible to reduce the error caused by the adjustment.

It should also be mentioned that the sole outcome parameter was the WRS at 65 dB; speech perception in noise and subjective hearing perception, e.g., music hearing, were not assessed. In further studies, one might investigate to what extent the position of the electrode array affects these other outcome parameters since a frequency mismatch could possibly be more important here.

5. Conclusions

Our results support the previously published model for predicting outcomes after cochlear implantation. WRS_{max} plays a more important part than WRS_{65}(HA), by allowing the prediction of the outcome of cochlear implantation. With the help of the prediction model, improved pre-operative counselling of patients on the expected outcome can be provided for patients with a pre-operative WRS_{max} greater than zero. For the implants used (CI622 and CI522) the insertion depth did not influence the post-operative outcome. The surgeon did not influence the outcome positively or negatively according to the distance (*d*) from the first electrode contact to the cochlear window within the observed range.

Author Contributions: Conceptualization, A.F.-T.; Methodology, A.F.-T.; Software, A.F.-T.; Validation, A.F.-T.; Formal analysis, A.F.-T.; Investigation, A.F.-T.; Data curation, A.F.-T., S.L., J.S. and K.M.; Writing—original draft, A.F.-T. and S.L.; Writing—review & editing, A.F.-T., S.L., T.Z. and M.N.; Visualization, A.F.-T.; Supervision, T.Z. and M.N.; Project administration, A.F.-T.; Funding acquisition, A.F.-T. and T.Z. All authors have read and agreed to the published version of the manuscript.

Funding: This research was funded by Cochlear Research & Development Ltd., (IIR2341).

Institutional Review Board Statement: This study was conducted in accordance with the Declaration of Helsinki and approved by the Institutional Ethics Committee of Technische Universität Dresden (SR+BO-260052021). The study was also registered under DRKS00026741 with the German register of clinical studies.

Informed Consent Statement: Informed consent was obtained from all subjects involved in the study.

Data Availability Statement: Supporting raw data may be obtained through special request from the corresponding author.

Conflicts of Interest: The authors declare no conflict of interest.

References

1. Buchman, C.A.; Gifford, R.H.; Haynes, D.S.; Lenarz, T.; O'Donoghue, G.; Adunka, O.; Biever, A.; Briggs, R.J.; Carlson, M.L.; Dai, P.; et al. Unilateral Cochlear Implants for Severe, Profound, or Moderate Sloping to Profound Bilateral Sensorineural Hearing Loss: A Systematic Review and Consensus Statements. *JAMA Otolaryngol. Head Neck Surg.* **2020**, *146*, 942–953. [CrossRef] [PubMed]
2. Blamey, P.J.; Artieres, F.; Baskent, D.; Bergeron, F.; Beynon, A.; Burke, E.; Dillier, N.; Dowell, R.; Fraysse, B.; Gallégo, S.; et al. Factors affecting auditory performance of postlinguistically deaf adults using cochlear implants: An update with 2251 patients. *Audiol. Neurotol.* **2013**, *18*, 36–47. [CrossRef] [PubMed]
3. Holden, L.K.; Finley, C.C.; Firszt, J.B.; Holden, T.A.; Brenner, C.; Potts, L.G.; Gotter, B.D.; Vanderhoof, S.S.; Mispagel, K.; Heydebrand, G.; et al. Factors affecting open-set word recognition in adults with cochlear implants. *Ear Hear.* **2013**, *34*, 342–360. [CrossRef] [PubMed]
4. Hoppe, U.; Hocke, T.; Hast, A.; Iro, H. Maximum preimplantation monosyllabic score as predictor of cochlear implant outcome. *HNO* **2019**, *67*, 62–68. [CrossRef] [PubMed]
5. Hoppe, U.; Hocke, T.; Hast, A.; Iro, H. Cochlear Implantation in Candidates with Moderate-to-Severe Hearing Loss and Poor Speech Perception. *Laryngoscope* **2021**, *131*, E940–E945. [CrossRef] [PubMed]
6. Goudey, B.; Plant, K.; Kiral, I.; Jimeno-Yepes, A.; Swan, A.; Gambhir, M.; Büchner, A.; Kludt, E.; Eikelboom, R.H.; Sucher, C.; et al. A MultiCenter Analysis of Factors Associated with Hearing Outcome for 2,735 Adults with Cochlear Implants. *Trends Hear.* **2021**, *25*, 23312165211037525. [CrossRef]
7. Shafieibavani, E.; Goudey, B.; Kiral, I.; Zhong, P.; Jimeno-Yepes, A.; Swan, A.; Gambhir, M.; Buechner, A.; Kludt, E.; Eikelboom, R.H.; et al. Predictive models for cochlear implant outcomes: Performance, generalizability, and the impact of cohort size. *Trends Hear.* **2021**, *25*, 23312165211066174. [CrossRef]
8. Thangavelu, K.; Nitzge, M.; Weiß, R.M.; Mueller-Mazzotta, J.; Stuck, B.A.; Reimann, K. Role of cochlear reserve in adults with cochlear implants following post-lingual hearing loss. *Eur. Arch. Otorhinolaryngol.* **2023**, *280*, 1063–1071. [CrossRef]
9. Hoppe, U.; Hast, A.; Hocke, T. Validation of a predictive model for speech discrimination after cochlear implant provision. *HNO* **2023**, *71*, 53–59. [CrossRef]

10. Franke-Trieger, A.; Jolly, C.; Darbinjan, A.; Zahnert, T.; Murbe, D. Insertion depth angles of cochlear implant arrays with varying length: A temporal bone study. *Otol. Neurotol.* **2014**, *35*, 58–63. [CrossRef]
11. Mewes, A.; Brademann, G.; Hey, M. Comparison of Perimodiolar Electrodes: Imaging and Electrophysiological Outcomes. *Otol. Neurotol.* **2020**, *41*, e934–e944. [CrossRef] [PubMed]
12. Liebscher, T.; Mewes, A.; Hoppe, U.; Hornung, J.; Brademann, G.; Hey, M. Electrode Translocations in Perimodiolar Cochlear Implant Electrodes: Audiological and Electrophysiological Outcome. *Z. Med. Phys.* **2021**, *31*, 265–275. [CrossRef] [PubMed]
13. Risi, F. Considerations and Rationale for Cochlear Implant Electrode Design—Past, Present and Future. *J. Int. Adv. Otol.* **2018**, *14*, 382–391. [CrossRef] [PubMed]
14. Dhanasingh, A. The rationale for FLEX (cochlear implant) electrode with varying array lengths. *World J. Otorhinolaryngol. Head Neck Surg.* **2021**, *7*, 45–53. [CrossRef] [PubMed]
15. Aniket, S.; Litvak, L.; Boyle, P. SPAN: Improved current steering on the Advanced Bionics CII and HiRes90K system. *Cochlear Implant. Int.* **2010**, *11*, 465–468.
16. Müller, A.; Hocke, T.; Mir-Salim, P. Intraoperative findings on ECAP-measurement: Normal or special case? *Int. J. Audiol.* **2015**, *54*, 257–264. [CrossRef] [PubMed]
17. Hoppe, U.; Brademann, G.; Stöver, T.; Ramos de Miguel, A.; Cowan, R.; Manrique, M.; Falcón-González, J.C.; Hey, M.; Baumann, U.; Huarte, A.; et al. Evaluation of a Transimpedance Matrix Algorithm to Detect Anomalous Cochlear Implant Electrode Position. *Audiol. Neurootol.* **2022**, *27*, 347–355. [CrossRef] [PubMed]
18. Aschendorff, A.; Kromeier, J.; Klenzner, T.; Laszig, R. Quality control after insertion of the nucleus contour and contour advance electrode in adults. *Ear Hear.* **2007**, *28*, 75S–79S. [CrossRef]
19. Basta, D.; Todt, I.; Ernst, A. Audiological outcome of the pull-back technique in cochlear implantees. *Laryngoscope* **2010**, *120*, 1391–1396. [CrossRef]
20. Riemann, C.; Sudhoff, H.; Todt, I. The Pull-Back Technique for the 532 Slim Modiolar Electrode. *Biomed Res. Int.* **2019**, *2019*, 6917084. [CrossRef]
21. Lailach, S.; Neudert, M.; Zahnert, T. Update cochlear-implantation: Indications and surgical aspects. *Laryngorhinootologie* **2021**, *100*, 652–672. [CrossRef] [PubMed]
22. Dziemba, O.C.; Merz, S.; Hocke, T. Evaluative audiometry after cochlear implant provision. *HNO* **2023**, *71*, 669–677. [CrossRef] [PubMed]
23. Winkler, A.; Holube, I. Test-retest reliability of the Freiburg monosyllabic speech test. *HNO* **2016**, *64*, 564–571. [CrossRef] [PubMed]
24. Verbist, B.M.; Skinner, M.W.; Cohen, L.T.; Leake, P.A.; James, C.; Boëx, C.; Holden, T.A.; Finley, C.C.; Roland, P.S.; Roland, J.T., Jr.; et al. Consensus panel on a cochlear coordinate system applicable in histological, physiological and radiological studies of the human cochlea. *Otol. Neurotol. Off. Publ. Am. Otol. Soc. Am. Neurotol. Soc. Eur. Acad. Otol. Neurotol.* **2010**, *31*, 722–730. [CrossRef] [PubMed]
25. Franke-Trieger, A.; Mürbe, D. Estimation of insertion depth angle based on cochlea diameter and linear insertion depth: A prediction tool for the CI422. *Eur. Arch. Otorhinolaryngol.* **2015**, *272*, 3193–3199. [CrossRef] [PubMed]
26. Rieck, J.H.; Beyer, A.; Mewes, A.; Caliebe, A.; Hey, M. Extended Preoperative Audiometry for Outcome Prediction and Risk Analysis in Patients Receiving Cochlear Implants. *J. Clin. Med.* **2023**, *12*, 3262. [CrossRef] [PubMed]
27. Franks, Z.G.; Jacob, A. The speech perception gap in cochlear implant patients. *Cochlear Implant. Int.* **2019**, *20*, 176–181. [CrossRef] [PubMed]
28. Hoppe, U.; Hast, A.; Hocke, T. Sprachverstehen mit Hörgeraten in Abhängigkeit vom Tongehör. *HNO* **2014**, *62*, 443–448. [CrossRef]
29. MacPhail, M.E.; Connell, N.T.; Totten, D.J.; Gray, M.T.; Pisoni, D.; Yates, C.W.; Nelson, R.F. Speech Recognition Outcomes in Adults with Slim Straight and Slim Modiolar Cochlear Implant Electrode Arrays. *Otolaryngol. Head Neck Surg.* **2022**, *166*, 943–950. [CrossRef]
30. Moran, M.; Vandali, A.; Briggs, R.J.S.; Dettman, S.; Cowan, R.S.C.; Dowell, R.C. Speech Perception Outcomes for Adult Cochlear Implant Recipients Using a Lateral Wall or Perimodiolar Array. *Otol. Neurotol.* **2019**, *40*, 608–616. [CrossRef]
31. Lauer, G.; Uçta, J.; Decker, L.; Ernst, A.; Mittmann, P. Intracochlear Pressure Changes After Cochlea Implant Electrode Pullback-Reduction of Intracochlear Trauma. *Laryngoscope Investig. Otolaryngol.* **2019**, *4*, 441–445. [CrossRef] [PubMed]
32. Cochlear Nucleus CI622 cochlear implant with slim straight electrode Physicians Guide CI622. Available online: https://mss-p-007-delivery.stylelabs.cloud/api/public/content/75f1036c47a44e88be373bc134305624?v=3a4edc74 (accessed on 27 December 2023).
33. Spiegel, J.L.; Polterauer, D.; Hempel, J.M.; Canis, M.; Spiro, J.E.; Müller, J. Variation of the cochlear anatomy and cochlea duct length: Analysis with a new tablet-based software. *Eur. Arch. Otorhinolaryngol.* **2022**, *279*, 1851–1861. [CrossRef] [PubMed]
34. Yukawa, K.; Cohen, L.; Blamey, P.; Pyman, B.; Tungvachirakul, V.; O'Leary, S. Effects of insertion depth of cochlear implant electrodes upon speech perception. *Audiol. Neurootol.* **2004**, *9*, 163–172. [CrossRef] [PubMed]
35. Fan, T.; Xiang, M.Y.; Li, Y.; Gong, J.M.; Wu, T.; Wang, Y.; Xu, J.; Wang, Y.F.; Li, J. Effect of Electrode Insertion Angle on Cochlear Implantation Outcomes in Adult and Children Patients with Sensorineural Hearing Loss. *Oxid. Med. Cell Longev.* **2022**, *2022*, 9914716. [CrossRef] [PubMed]

36. Canfarotta, M.W.; Dillon, M.T.; Brown, K.D.; Pillsbury, H.C.; Dedmon, M.M.; O'Connell, B.P. Insertion Depth and Cochlear Implant Speech Recognition Outcomes: A Comparative Study of 28- and 31.5-mm Lateral Wall Arrays. *Otol. Neurotol.* **2022**, *43*, 183–189. [CrossRef] [PubMed]
37. Roßberg, C.; Timm, M.; Roßberg, W.; Kludt, E.; Bronzlik, P.; Lesinski-Schiedat, A.; Büchner, A.; Lenarz, T. Comparison of speech understanding taking into account the exact electrode position (SRA/MRA/CA). *Laryngorhinootologie* **2023**, *102*, 850–855. [CrossRef] [PubMed]
38. Ketterer, M.C.; Aschendorff, A.; Arndt, S.; Beck, R. Electrode array design determines scalar position, dislocation rate and angle and postoperative speech perception. *Eur. Arch. Otorhinolaryngol.* **2022**, *279*, 4257–4267. [CrossRef] [PubMed]
39. Thimsen, V.; Mantsopoulos, K.; Liebscher, T.; Taha, L.; Eisenhut, F.; Iro, H.; Hoppe, U.; Hornung, J. Association between lateral wall electrode array insertion parameters and audiological outcomes in bilateral cochlear implantation. *Eur. Arch. Otorhinolaryngol.* **2023**, *280*, 2707–2714. [CrossRef]
40. Başkent, D.; Shannon, R.V. Interactions between cochlear implant electrode insertion depth and frequency-place mapping. *J. Acoust. Soc. Am.* **2005**, *117*, 1405–1416. [CrossRef]
41. Finley, C.C.; Holden, T.A.; Holden, L.K.; Whiting, B.R.; Chole, R.A.; Neely, G.J.; Hullar, T.E.; Skinner, M.W. Role of electrode placement as a contributor to variability in cochlear implant outcomes. *Otol. Neurotol.* **2008**, *29*, 920–928. [CrossRef]
42. Heutink, F.; de Rijk, S.R.; Verbist, B.M.; Huinck, W.J.; Mylanus, E.A.M. Angular Electrode Insertion Depth and Speech Perception in Adults with a Cochlear Implant: A Systematic Review. *Otol. Neurotol.* **2019**, *40*, 900–910. [CrossRef]
43. Faulkner, A.; Rosen, S.; Norman, C. The right information may matter more than frequency-place alignment: Simulations of frequency-aligned and upward shifting cochlear implant processors for a shallow electrode array insertion. *Ear Hear.* **2006**, *27*, 139–152. [CrossRef] [PubMed]
44. Suhling, M.C.; Majdani, O.; Salcher, R.; Leifholz, M.; Buchner, A.; Lesinski-Schiedat, A.; Lenarz, T. The Impact of Electrode Array Length on Hearing Preservation in Cochlear Implantation. *Otol. Neurotol.* **2016**, *37*, 1006–1015. [CrossRef]
45. Mewes, A.; Burg, S.; Brademann, G.; Dambon, J.A.; Hey, M. Quality-assured training in the evaluation of cochlear implant electrode position: A prospective experimental study. *BMC Med. Educ.* **2022**, *22*, 386. [CrossRef] [PubMed]
46. Böttcher-Rebmann, G.; Schell, V.; Zuniga, M.G.; Salcher, R.; Lenarz, T.; Rau, T.S. Preclinical evaluation of a tool for insertion force measurements in cochlear implant surgery. *Int. J. Comput. Assist. Radiol. Surg.* **2023**, *18*, 2117–2124. [CrossRef] [PubMed]
47. Van der Jagt, A.M.A.; Briaire, J.J.; Boehringer, S.; Verbist, B.M.; Frijns, J.H.M. Prolonged Insertion Time Reduces Translocation Rate of a Precurved Electrode Array in Cochlear Implantation. *Otol. Neurotol.* **2022**, *43*, e427–e434. [CrossRef]
48. Barriat, S.; Peigneux, N.; Duran, U.; Camby, S.; Lefebvre, P.P. The Use of a Robot to Insert an Electrode Array of Cochlear Implants in the Cochlea: A Feasibility Study and Preliminary Results. *Audiol. Neurootol.* **2021**, *26*, 361–367. [CrossRef]
49. Lenarz, T.; Buechner, A.; Gantz, B.; Hansen, M.; Tejani, V.D.; Labadie, R.; O'Connell, B.; Buchman, C.A.; Valenzuela, C.V.; Adunka, O.F.; et al. Relationship Between Intraoperative Electrocochleography and Hearing Preservation. *Otol. Neurotol.* **2022**, *43*, e72–e78. [CrossRef]
50. Arweiler-Harbeck, D.; D'Heygere, V.; Meyer, M.; Hans, S.; Waschkies, L.; Lang, S.; Anton, K.; Hessel, H.; Schneider, A.; Heiler, T.; et al. Digital Live Imaging of Intraoperative Electrocochleography—First Description of Feasibility and Hearing Preservation during Cochlear Implantation. *Otol. Neurotol.* **2021**, *42*, 1342–1346. [CrossRef]
51. Harrison, L.; Manjaly, J.G.; Ellis, W.; Lavy, J.A.; Shaida, A.; Khalil, S.S.; Saeed, S.R. Hearing Preservation Outcomes with Standard Length Electrodes in Adult Cochlear Implantation and the Uptake of Electroacoustic Stimulation. *Otol. Neurotol.* **2020**, *41*, 1060–1065. [CrossRef]
52. Spitzer, E.R.; Waltzman, S.B.; Landsberger, D.M.; Friedmann, D.R. Acceptance and Benefits of Electro-Acoustic Stimulation for Conventional-Length Electrode Arrays. *Audiol. Neurootol.* **2021**, *26*, 17–26. [CrossRef] [PubMed]
53. Van de Heyning, P.H.; Dazert, S.; Gavilan, J.; Lassaletta, L.; Lorens, A.; Rajan, G.P.; Skarzynski, H.; Skarzynski, P.H.; Tavora-Vieira, D.; Topsakal, V.; et al. Systematic Literature Review of Hearing Preservation Rates in Cochlear Implantation Associated with Medium- and Longer-Length Flexible Lateral Wall Electrode Arrays. *Front. Surg.* **2022**, *9*, 893839. [CrossRef] [PubMed]
54. Dalbert, A.; Huber, A.; Baumann, N.; Veraguth, D.; Roosli, C.; Pfiffner, F. Hearing Preservation After Cochlear Implantation May Improve Long-term Word Perception in the Electric-only Condition. *Otol. Neurotol.* **2016**, *37*, 1314–1319. [CrossRef] [PubMed]
55. Buchner, A.; Illg, A.; Majdani, O.; Lenarz, T. Investigation of the effect of cochlear implant electrode length on speech comprehension in quiet and noise compared with the results with users of electro-acoustic-stimulation, a retrospective analysis. *PLoS ONE* **2017**, *12*, e0174900. [CrossRef]
56. Rader, T.; Doms, P.; Adel, Y.; Weissgerber, T.; Strieth, S.; Baumann, U. A method for determining precise electrical hearing thresholds in cochlear implant users. *Int. J. Audiol.* **2018**, *57*, 502–509. [CrossRef]
57. Plesch, J.; Ernst, B.P.; Strieth, S.; Rader, T. A psychoacoustic application for the adjustment of electrical hearing thresholds in cochlear implant patients. *PLoS ONE* **2019**, *14*, e0223625. [CrossRef]

Journal of
Clinical Medicine

MDPI

Article

Impact of Reverberation on Speech Perception in Noise in Bimodal/Bilateral Cochlear Implant Users with and without Residual Hearing

Clara König [1,*], Uwe Baumann [1], Timo Stöver [2] and Tobias Weissgerber [1]

1 Audiological Acoustics, ENT Department, University Hospital, Goethe University Frankfurt, 60590 Frankfurt am Main, Germany; uwe.baumann@unimedizin-ffm.de (U.B.); weissgerber@med.uni-frankfurt.de (T.W.)

2 ENT Department, University Hospital, Goethe University Frankfurt, 60590 Frankfurt am Main, Germany; stoever@med.uni-frankfurt.de

* Correspondence: clara.koenig@unimedizin-ffm.de; Tel.: +49-151-17191140

Abstract: (1) **Background**: The aim of the present study was to assess the impact of reverberation on speech perception in noise and spatial release from masking (SRM) in bimodal or bilateral cochlear implant (CI) users and CI subjects with low-frequency residual hearing using combined electric–acoustic stimulation (EAS). (2) **Methods**: In total, 10 bimodal, 14 bilateral CI users and 14 EAS users, and 17 normal hearing (NH) controls, took part in the study. Speech reception thresholds (SRTs) in unmodulated noise were assessed in co-located masker condition (S0N0) with a spatial separation of speech and noise (S0N60) in both free-field and loudspeaker-based room simulation for two different reverberation times. (3) **Results**: There was a significant detrimental effect of reverberation on SRTs and SRM in all subject groups. A significant difference between the NH group and all the CI/EAS groups was found. There was no significant difference in SRTs between any CI and EAS group. Only NH subjects achieved spatial release from masking in reverberation, whereas no beneficial effect of spatial separation of speech and noise was found in any CI/EAS group. (4) **Conclusions**: The subject group with electric–acoustic stimulation did not yield a superior outcome in terms of speech perception in noise under reverberation when the noise was presented towards the better hearing ear.

Keywords: cochlear implant; electric–acoustic stimulation; reverberation; speech perception; spatial release from masking

1. Introduction

Cochlear implants (CIs) can help many users with severe to profound sensorineural hearing loss to achieve good speech perception in quiet within a range that is often comparable to that of individuals with normal hearing (NH) [1]. However, CI users oftentimes struggle to understand speech in everyday listening conditions that comprise noise sources and/or reverberation [2,3].

For NH listeners, speech perception in noisy environments improves when the signal and noise sources are spatially separated compared to co-located speech and masker conditions. This effect is called spatial release from masking (SRM) which is primarily caused by binaural (i.e., spatial) hearing (interaural level differences and interaural time differences) in combination with monaural better ear effects [4,5]. Previous studies have shown that the improvement in speech perception using SRM is reduced or even absent in bilateral CI users or bimodal CI users using a hearing aid in the contralateral ear [6,7].

Another effect which deteriorates speech perception in NH as well as in CI users is reverberation. While speech perception in quiet is hardly affected by reverberation in people with normal hearing, there is a significant reduction in speech perception in cochlear implant users [2,8–10]. On the other hand, it was reported that reverberation has comparable detrimental effects on speech perception in noise for both NH and CI subjects [11,12]. However, it has to be noted that CI users are by far more affected by reverberation in everyday life since their performance (measured as speech reception threshold, SRT, measured in dB SNR) in the free-field is already up to 10 dB worse than in NH [11]. Studies investigating the effect of reverberation on speech perception in CI users were oftentimes conducted in simulated reverberation via headphone presentation or by using the direct audio input of the CI [3,8,10,13–15]. Furthermore, oftentimes CI listening with vocoder simulation instead of testing real CI subjects was performed [2,7,8,10,13–17].

Only a few studies investigated the effect of reverberation on speech perception in CI recipients using a real sound field by means of a loudspeaker array, allowing every tested person to use their individual head-related transfer functions [11,12,18]. It was shown that the impact of reverberation on SRTs in CI users was weaker than in studies using less complex room simulation methods without real loudspeakers. Therefore, the aim of the present study was to compare the impact of reverberation on speech perception in noise and SRM for different groups of CI users with and without residual hearing in one or both ears in a loudspeaker-based sound reproduction setup.

A special focus will be placed here on the group with combined electric–acoustic stimulation (EAS), which has been insufficiently studied in the past since many of the aforementioned studies only compared speech perception performance between NH listeners, bimodal CI listeners and bilateral CI listeners. EAS is a well-accepted therapeutic treatment for CI users with residual hearing in the low frequencies but severe to profound hearing loss in the high frequencies [19]. The unilateral combination of the electric stimulation of the high frequencies via a CI and acoustic stimulation of the low frequencies via a hearing aid enables users to achieve better speech perception in quiet [20,21], in noise [20–26], and better sound localisation [26,27] than electric-only stimulation does. It is assumed that the benefit of the EAS listeners comes from access to frequency fine structure and F0 information, which facilitates the identification of low-frequency acoustic landmarks such as the onset of voicing and the syllable structure [28,29]. In a study with simulated CI and EAS listening, the largest SRM that was closest to the NH listeners was found in the group of bilateral EAS users [7]. To the knowledge of the authors, no studies comparing speech perception in reverberation between CI and EAS in loudspeaker-based sound reproduction setups have been published so far.

2. Materials and Methods

2.1. Subject Demographics

A total of 10 unilateral CI users with a hearing aid in the contralateral ear (i.e., bimodal CI users; 6 female, mean age: 52.5 ± 19.2 years), 14 bilateral CI users (8 female, mean age: 49.9 ± 16.4 years) and two groups of EAS users (bimodal group with hearing aid or CI in contralateral ear: n = 8, 5 female, mean age: 60.1 ± 8.5 years; bilateral group: n = 6, 3 female, mean age: 61.5 ± 12.4 years) took part in the study. All participants were implanted with MED-EL (Innsbruck, Austria) devices with either SONNET or OPUS 2 (or DUET 2 for EAS) sound processors. The minimum experience with their CI was 2.4 months and the mean duration of cochlear implant use was 5.2 years, ranging from 2.4 months to 17.4 years. The inclusion criterion was that the individual monosyllable score in quiet (Freiburg monosyllables at 65 dB sound pressure level, [30]) and in the ipsilateral ear (or in cases with bilateral CI/EAS in the better hearing ear) had to be better than 50%. For lower speech perception scores in quiet, no measurement of speech reception thresholds in noise would be feasible. All subjects were tested with their everyday fitting map. The proper fitting of sound processors and hearing aids was assessed using aided free-field audiometry (hearing thresholds) and speech audiometry (Freiburg monosyllable score). In case of the use of the SONNET sound processor, the microphone directionality was set to omnidirectional. Detailed information on all CI/EAS users can be found in Tables 1–4.

Table 1. Data of the bimodal subject group. FMS: Freiburg monosyllable score. PTA: pure-tone average of frequencies 0.5/1/2/4 kHz. Used hearing aids were from manufacturers Unitron (Kitchener, ON, Canada), Phonak (Stäfa, Switzerland), Audio Service (Löhne, Germany), ReSound (Ballerup, Denmark), and Widex (Lynge, Denmark).

ID	Implant Type (Ear)	Age [yrs]	Sound Processor	CI Listening Experience [yrs]	Hearing Aid Type	FMS CI [%]	FMS HA [%]	PTA (Contralateral) [dB HL]
BM 1	Concerto Flex24 (right)	57.3	OPUS 2	4.2	Unitron Moda 2	95	95	35.0
BM 2	Concerto Flex24 (right)	73.6	OPUS 2	3.6	Phonak Dalia SC	75	25	88.8
BM 3	Pulsar Standard (left)	23.6	OPUS 2	16.3	Phonak Naida S	90	0	106.3
BM 4	Concerto Flex28 (right)	71.9	OPUS 2	4.3	Phonak Naida S3	55	85	47.5
BM 5	Synchrony Flex28 (left)	67.6	SONNET	2.2	Audio Service Mezzo Duo	70	0	77.5
BM 6	Synchrony Flex28 (left)	34.7	SONNET	2.0	ReSound Preza	80	40	103.8
BM 7	Concerto Flex28 (left)	73.0	OPUS 2	5.0	Phonak Naida S V UP	85	55	77.5
BM 8	Synchrony Flex28 (left)	33.0	OPUS 2	2.1	Phonak Naida 5 S1	65	60	61.3
BM 9	Sonata Flex24 (right)	55.2	OPUS 2	7.1	Widex Inteo	60	30	101.3
BM 10	Synchrony Flex28 (left)	35.7	SONNET	1.6	Phonak Naida Q50-SP	80	80	43.8

Table 2. Data of the bilateral subject group. FMS: Freiburg monosyllable score, ipsilateral ear for noise presentation in S0N60 test condition is indicated bold.

ID	Implant Type (Left/Right)	Age [yrs]	Sound Processor	CI Listening Experience Left [yrs]	CI Listening Experience Right [yrs]	FMS Left [%]	FMS Right [%]
BL 1	Concerto Flex28/FlexSoft	63.3	OPUS 2	4.1	5.2	70	**85**
BL 2	Concerto FLEXsoft/FLEX28	57.6	OPUS 2	5.0	4.0	**95**	95
BL 3	Concerto FLEXsoft/FLEX28	70.1	OPUS 2	4.2	5.4	**85**	85
BL 4	Sonata FLEXsoft Pulsar Standard	50.1	OPUS 2	6.3	9.9	**90**	80
BL 5	Concerto FLEX24	59.5	OPUS 2	3.7	2.9	75	**80**
BL 6	Concerto FLEX28 C40+ Standard	38.1	OPUS 2	4.4	13.6	85	**90**
BL 7	Sonata Standard Sonata FLEXsoft	65.7	OPUS 2	8.7	6.2	**80**	55
BL 8	Concerto FLEX28	47.1	OPUS 2	3.4	3.4	**75**	65
BL 9	Concerto FLEX28	27.3	OPUS 2	3.6	2.3	**90**	35
BL 10	C40+ Standard	30.0	SONNET	14.4	14.6	**100**	100
BL 11	Synchrony FLEX28 Concerto FLEX28	63.2	OPUS 2/SONNET	1.0	3.6	60	**80**
BL 12	C40+ Standard	19.2	OPUS 2	15.3	17.4	**95**	85
BL 13	Concerto FLEX28	41.5	OPUS 2	3.9	3.9	**80**	70
BL 14	Concerto FLEX28	66.3	OPUS 2/SONNET	2.0	3.6	80	**95**

Table 3. Data of the bimodal EAS group. FMS: Freiburg monosyllable score. PTA: pure-tone average of frequencies 0.5/1/2/4 kHz. PTA_{low}: pure-tone average of frequencies 125/250/500 Hz. Used hearing aids were from manufacturers Phonak (Stäfa, Switzerland, Oticon (Smørum, Denmark), and Siemens (Erlangen, Germany).

ID	Implant Type (Ear)	Age [yrs]	Sound Processor	EAS Listening Experience [yrs]	Hearing Aid Type	FMS Score EAS/Contra [%]	PTA EAS/Contra [dB HL]	PTA_{low} EAS [dB HL]
EAS_BM1	Sonata FLEX24 (left)	55.8	SONNET EAS	5.3	Phonak Naida S IX UP	70/70	117.5/81.3	73.3
EAS_BM2	Sonata FLEX24 (right)	53.5	SONNET EAS	5.8	Phonak Piconet 2 P2 AZ	85/20	102.5/101.3	43.3
EAS_BM3	Sonata FLEX20 (right)	73.8	SONNET EAS	5.9	SONNET (CI)	65/55	86.3/94	61.7
EAS_BM4	Synchrony FLEX24 (left)	70.8	SONNET EAS	2.0	Oticon Chili SP9	70/30	82.5/76	71.7
EAS_BM5	Synchrony FLEX24 (right)	59.7	SONNET EAS	4.1	SONNET (CI)	85/80	107.5/120	53.3
EAS_BM6	Concerto FLEX24 (right)	63.4	SONNET EAS	4.4	Siemens Nitro	95/35	98.8/84	38.3
EAS_BM7	Sonata FLEX24 (right)	52.7	SONNET EAS	6.8	-	85/25	101.3/110	31.7
EAS_BM8	Concerto FLEX24 (right)	51.3	OPUS 2 EAS	4.1	Siemens Motion P	50/30	98.8/98	51.7

Table 4. Data of the bilateral EAS group. FMS: Freiburg monosyllable score; ipsilateral ear for noise presentation in S0N60 test condition is indicated bold. PTA: pure-tone average of frequencies 0.5/1/2/4 kHz. PTA_{low}: pure-tone average of frequencies 125/250/500 Hz.

ID	Implant Type (Left/Right)	Age [yrs]	Sound Processor (Left/Right)	EAS Listening Experience Left [yrs]	EAS Listening Experience Right [yrs]	FMS Score Left/Right [%]	PTA L/R [dB HL]	PTA_{low} L/R [dB HL]
EAS_BL1	Synchrony FLEX24	72.9	SONNET EAS	1.1	1.9	**100**/80	106.3/93.8	66.7/46.7
EAS_BL2	Sonata FLEX20/FLEX24	73.9	OPUS 2 EAS	6.2	7.6	70/**80**	106.3/100	85/73.3
EAS_BL3	Sonata FLEX24 Synchrony FLEX24	60.5	DUET 2 SONNET EAS	5.1	1.1	**85**/70	120/108.8	81.7/48.3
EAS_BL4	Concerto FLEX24	47.8	SONNET EAS	2.6	4.2	**100**/70	77.5/106.3	16.7/53.3
EAS_BL5	Concerto FLEX24 Sonata FLEX24	68.1	DUET 2 SONNET EAS	3.6	5.0	**75**/65	112.5/111.3	68.3/56.6
EAS_BL6	Synchrony FLEX24	45.6	SONNET EAS	0.2	0.3	**90**/80	106.3/88.8	23.3/21.7

A group of 17 subjects (14 female, mean age: 26.7 ± 8.0 years) with normal hearing (i.e., no pure-tone hearing loss >25 dB HL in any test frequency between 0.125 and 8 kHz) served as a control group.

2.2. Speech Perception Test in Reverberation

Testing was performed in an anechoic chamber using 128 custom-built loudspeakers which were mounted in the horizontal plane at a height of 1.20 m. The distance between adjacent loudspeakers was 8.6 cm. Further information about the loudspeakers setup is given in [31]. Speech tests were conducted in free-field conditions and under loudspeaker-based reverberation simulation. Reverberation was created with a custom room simulation tool combining the nearest speaker method for early reflections and a feedback delay network to simulate late reflections [32]. For the room simulation in the present study, a three-dimensional model of a lecture hall simulated with two different degrees of absorption corresponding to reverberation times of 0.35 s and 0.51 s was used [32].

Speech perception in noise was measured with the German Matrix Test (Oldenburg Sentence Test, OlSa, [33]). The noise level was kept constant at 65 dB SPL. The speech level was adaptively changed to measure the speech reception threshold (SRT) for a 50% correct word understanding. The speech signal was always presented from frontal direction (0° azimuth). The noise signal was the continuous noise of the OlSa test which was either presented from the front (i.e., co-located masker at 0°, S0N0) or from the side (either from +60° or −60° azimuth, S0N60). In the S0N60 condition, the noise was always presented on the side of the CI/EAS system in the case of bimodal CI/EAS users or on the side of the better ear in the case of bilateral CI/EAS fitting. Both spatial configurations of S0N0 and S0N60 were tested in free-field and in reverberation with 0.35 s and 0.51 s reverberation time, respectively. One OlSa list with 20 sentences each was used for each test condition. Prior to testing, one practice list was presented to the subject to familiarise the subject with the test procedure and the speech material. The test was conducted in a closed-set mode and the order of the test lists was randomised.

All study tests in this prospective study were performed for each subject on a single appointment. The test duration was approximately 90–120 min.

2.3. Statistics

Boxplots and median values were used for descriptive analyses throughout the manuscript. Nonparametric tests were utilised for statistical analyses of SRT differences (group differences: Kruskal–Wallis H test; impact of test condition within subject groups: Friedman test). Post hoc tests were performed using the Mann–Whitney U-test (group differences) or the Wilcoxon test (within-group). Correlations were tested via Spearman rank correlation. A p value < 0.05 was considered significant. IBM SPSS Statistics 27 (IBM, Armonik, New York, NY, USA) was used for the analysis.

3. Results

3.1. Impact of Reverberation on SRTs

The boxplots of the SRT measurement results in the S0N0 condition in free-field and reverberation are shown for all participants in Figure 1. There was a significant effect of reverberation in all subject groups (NH: $X^2 = 28.4$, $p < 0.001$; CI bimodal: $X^2 = 20.0$, $p < 0.001$; CI bilateral: $X^2 = 23.3$, $p < 0.001$; EAS bimodal: $X^2 = 8.9$, $p = 0.012$; EAS bilateral: $X^2 = 10.3$, $p = 0.006$; all df = 2; Friedman test) showing higher SRTs with increasing reverberation time. The median SRT difference between the free-field condition and test condition with the highest reverberation time was between 2.2 dB (bilateral EAS group) and 3.4 dB (bimodal CI group).

There was also a significant effect of subject group on SRTs (free-field: H = 35.5; 0.35 s reverberation: H = 36.3; 0.51 s reverberation: H = 37.2; all $p < 0.001$; all df = 4; Kruskal–Wallis H test). Non-parametric post hoc tests found significant differences in SRT between the NH group and all CI/EAS groups (all $p < 0.001$). The SRTs in the NH group were 4.2–5.2 dB better than the SRTs in the CI and EAS groups. However, no significant difference in the SRTs was found between any CI/EAS group in test condition S0N0.

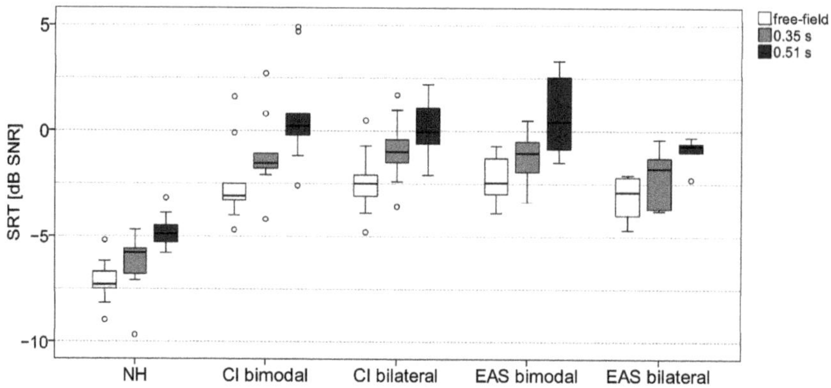

Figure 1. Boxplots of the SRT measurement results for all five subject groups in the S0N0 condition in free-field (white boxes) and reverberation with reverberation time of 0.35 s (light grey boxes) and 0.51 s (dark grey boxes). Each outlier that is more than 1.5 times the interquartile range is indicated with a circle.

The boxplots of the SRT measurements in the S0N60 condition of all participants in free-field and reverberation are shown in Figure 2. There was a significant effect of reverberation in all subject groups (NH: $X^2 = 30.5$, $p < 0.001$; CI bimodal: $X^2 = 18.2$, $p < 0.001$; CI bilateral: $X^2 = 26.1$, $p < 0.001$; EAS bimodal: $X^2 = 14.0$, $p < 0.001$; EAS bilateral: $X^2 = 12.0$, $p = 0.002$; all df = 2). The SRTs increased with increasing reverberation time. The median SRT difference between the free-field condition and test condition with the longest reverberation time was between 4.9 dB (bilateral EAS group) and 7.6 dB (bimodal CI group).

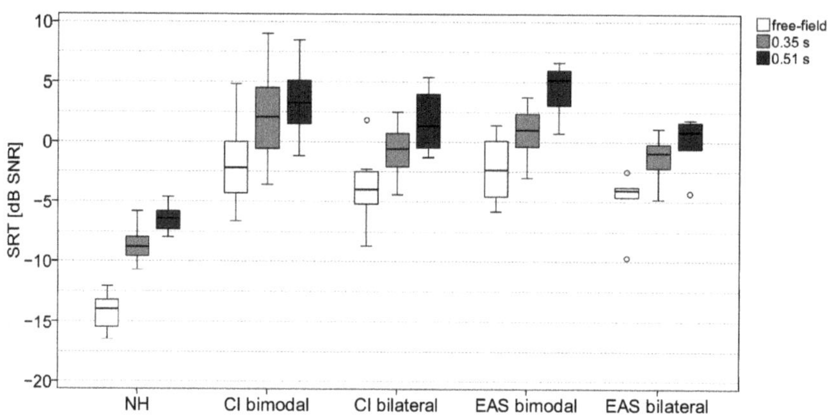

Figure 2. Boxplots of the SRT measurement results for all five subject groups in the S0N60 condition in free-field (white boxes) and reverberation with reverberation time of 0.35 s (light grey boxes) and 0.51 s (dark grey boxes). Each outlier that is more than 1.5 times the interquartile range is indicated with a circle.

There was also a significant effect of subject group on SRTs (free-field: H = 36.5, $p < 0.001$; 0.35 s reverberation: H = 37.7, $p < 0.001$; 0.51 s reverberation: H = 40.1, $p < 0.001$). Post hoc tests found significant differences in SRT between the NH group and all the CI/EAS groups (all $p < 0.001$). The SRTs in the NH group were 7.2–11.8 dB better than the SRTs in the CI and EAS groups. This was the same as the condition S0N0; no significant difference in SRTs was found between any CI and EAS group in test condition S0N60.

3.2. Impact of Reverberation on Spatial Release from Masking

The boxplots of spatial release from masking (SRM, i.e., individual SRT difference between S0N0 and S0N60) are shown in Figure 3. There was a significant effect of reverberation on SRM in the NH group ($X^2 = 30.2$, $p < 0.001$), the bimodal groups with CI ($X^2 = 13.3$, $p = 0.001$) and EAS ($X^2 = 14.3$, $p = 0.001$), and in the bilateral groups with CI ($X^2 = 9.0$, $p = 0.011$) and EAS ($X^2 = 12.3$, $p = 0.002$).

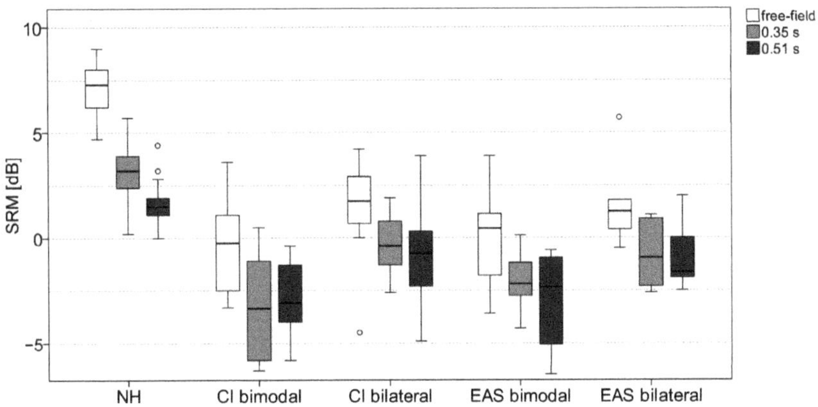

Figure 3. Boxplots of spatial release from masking (SRM, individual SRT difference between S0N0 and S0N60 results) for all five subject groups in free-field (white boxes) and reverberation with reverberation time of 0.35 s (light grey boxes) and 0.51 s (dark grey boxes). Each outlier that is more than 1.5 times the interquartile range is indicated with a circle.

There was also a significant effect of subject group on the SRM (free-field: $H = 37.6$, $p < 0.001$; 0.35 s reverberation: $H = 38.9$, $p < 0.001$; 0.51 s reverberation: $H = 30.3$, $p < 0.001$). Post hoc tests found significant differences in SRM between the NH group and all CI/EAS groups (all $p < 0.001$). SRM in the NH group was 2.3–7.6 dB higher than SRM in the CI and EAS groups.

No significant difference in SRM was found between any CI and EAS group. It should be noted, that only in the bilateral CI and EAS groups, the majority of subjects could benefit from a spatial separation of speech in noise to improve speech perception (but only under free-field conditions). In contrast, approximately 50% of subjects in the bimodal groups had no SRM at all (i.e., a SRM score lower or equal 0 dB).

3.3. Impact of Acoustic Hearing on SRT and SRM

For the bimodal CI and EAS groups, correlations were calculated between the pure-tone average (PTA, frequencies 0.5/1/2/4 kHz) or the low-frequency pure-tone average (PTA_{low}, frequencies 0.125/0.25/0.5 kHz) and SRT/SRM scores. There was no significant correlation between PTA or PTA_{low} and SRT or SRM scores in any subject group.

4. Discussion

4.1. Impact of Reverberation on SRTs

All subject groups showed a deterioration in SRTs in continuous noise with increasing reverberation time in both co-located S0N0 and spatially separated S0N60 conditions assessed in a loudspeaker-based room simulation setup. The detrimental effect of reverberation on SRT was 2.2–3.4 dB in the S0N0 condition and 4.9–7.6 dB in the S0N60 condition, depending on subject group. The detrimental effect of reverberation on SRTs was comparable in all subject groups. However, the baseline (i.e., SRT in free-field) was considerably higher (worse) in all CI groups, especially in the S0N60 condition (up to 12 dB).

To the knowledge of the authors, this is the first study that assessed the impact of reverberation on SRTs in noise in a population of EAS in comparison with the NH and CI groups using a loudspeaker-based sound reproduction setup. Helms-Tillery et al. investigated the effect of reverberation on speech perception in EAS using vocoder studies in NH subjects [17]. They found a significant "EAS effect" (better speech perception) in reverberation compared to simulated CI.

Kokkinakis and Loizou [8] reported for CI users a decrease in word recognition from 84% in an anechoic condition to 20% in reverberation (reverberation time: 1.0 s) at a source–receiver distance of 1 m. Kokkinakis et al. [34] extended this study by various reverberation times. They found that mean word recognition performance decreased exponentially with increasing reverberation time. In the present study, the relationship between reverberation time and SRT was rather linear. It must be taken into account that the method of room simulation differs significantly in many of the studies. Kokkinakis et al. used the static filtering of non-individualised head-related transfer functions (i.e., binaural and headphone based approach). Differences in sound reproduction could have a higher impact on the results. Many studies did not take place in a real room or loudspeaker-based room simulation, but were presented via a direct audio output (e.g., [8,10,13–15,34]), or, the participants did not wear their own processors but research processors, which may have varied from their everyday processor (e.g., [8,13,15,34]). It is assumed that by using the user's everyday CI system in a real sound field, more realistic spatial cues and natural reverberation can be included to reach results closer to real-life situations.

It should also be considered that reverberation is not the only room-acoustic parameter. In the present study, the reverberation time was modulated by changing the absorption properties of the surfaces inside the room while keeping the room geometry and the source and listener positions constant. Therefore, an increase in reverberation time goes along with a decrease in the direct-to-reverberant energy ratio (DRR). This means that the level of reverberation in relation to the direct sound is also increased. Thus, there were two acoustic parameters which could account for the deterioration in SRT.

In a real room, the reverberation time is almost place-independent, whereas the DRR is defined by the distance between source and listener. The influence of the distance between the talker and CI users was investigated by Kressner et al. [12] in a loudspeaker-based reproduction setup with three different room sizes and different receiver positions (1 m, 3 m, 6 m). They found a significant effect of the source–receiver distance, but no effect of the reverberation time on speech perception. Furthermore, no effect of the number of late reflections on speech perception was found. For a small source–receiver distance of 1 m (i.e., high DRRs), all participants except one showed speech perception scores better than 90%, even in a simulation of a large room (reverberation time: 1.7 s). These results contradict the data of Kokkinakis and Loizou [8] and Kokkinakis et al. [34], with a high impact of reverberation also at a small source–receiver distance, but measured with a binaural sound reproduction method. In the model of Kressner et al., an effect became significant with a source–receiver distance of 3 m and particularly worse in the big room auditorium simulation with a source-receiver distance of 6 m.

Badajoz-Davila et al. [18] also reported that speech perception does not necessarily decay with increasing reverberation time. The data were also obtained using loudspeaker-based sound reproduction. Speech perception in a smaller but more reflective room (reverberation time: 1.55 s) was more affected than in a bigger room (car park) with a higher reverberation time of 2.42 s. Badajoz-Davila et al. [18] assume that the quite strong effect of reverberation on speech perception in CI users that was observed in previous studies [2,3,8,14,34] is caused since small reverberant rooms were considered, containing an unrealistically high amount of reverberation.

In the present study, results close to everyday performance were expected since loudspeaker-based room simulation was used, which was shown to be beneficial compared to binaural sound reproduction methods in CI users. However, further studies should also assess the effect of DRR and reverberation time independently.

4.2. Impact of Reverberation on Spatial Release from Masking

Spatial release from masking as the effect of spatial separation of speech and continuous noise (measured as SRT difference between S0N0 and S0N60) was investigated for free-field conditions and two different reverberation times. In contrast to other studies, the separation was only 60° (i.e., no maximum head shadow effect as for 90°) and the noise was presented to the better hearing ear. A significant effect of reverberation on SRM was found for all subject groups. However, it has to be noted that even in free-field conditions, considerable differences in SRM between NH and all CI groups were found. The mean SRM in the NH group was higher than 7 dB, whereas in the bilateral CI and EAS groups only 75% of the subjects had a small SRM at all (median: 1.25–1.75 dB). In the bimodal groups, only 50% of the subjects achieved a small SRM in free-field conditions. No beneficial effect of EAS use on SRM was found.

The results are in line with data from Gifford et al. (2014). They found no beneficial effect of hearing preservation on SRM [6]. As in our study, the highest amount of SRM was in the bilateral CI group. Williges et al. [7] used vocoder studies to assess SRM in simulated CI and EAS subjects. SRM in the bilateral CI group was about 6 dB lower than in NH, which is in line with the data presented in our study. In contrast to the present results and the data reported in Gifford et al., a beneficial effect of EAS on SRM compared to bilateral CI was found.

SRM was severely deteriorated by reverberation in the NH group, showing decreasing SRM with increasing reverberation time. Rennies and Kidd [35] found that increasing reverberation not only leads to decreased SRM, but also to a strong deterioration of spatial release from listening effort.

None of the EAS or CI groups achieved any SRM in reverberation at all. The reason is probably that the noise was presented to the better ear. Since the subjects could benefit from the head shadow effect only in the poorer ear, SRM was already small in the free-field. By increasing diffusiveness due to reverberation, the head shadow effect was further diminished. It could be hypothesised that SRM in CI or EAS users would be higher in a symmetric noise/reverberation setup, where the better ear effect would be useable. The study of Weissgerber et al. [36] investigated SRM in a symmetric diffuse noise condition, showing that SRM in bimodal and the bilateral CI groups was comparable (2.1–2.2 dB) and close to NH (2.9 dB).

It has to be noted that the noise used in the present study was continuous noise. Further studies using temporally modulated noise were of interest to assess the combined effect of glimpsing and SRM in EAS vs. electric CI stimulation only.

4.3. Impact of Subject Group

There was a significant effect of subject group in all test conditions. However, post hoc tests revealed that only the results from the NH group were significantly different (i.e., better) compared to all EAS/CI groups, whereas no significant differences between the EAS or CI subject groups were found in any test condition.

These findings are in contradiction to other previous studies. The average EAS benefit in free-field is reported to be in the range of 5% to 30% in quiet [37] and 26% in noise [38]. Rader et al. [25] compared bilateral CI users and bimodal EAS users in the co-located masker condition S0N0 and in a diffuse multi-source noise field condition. In all test conditions, the EAS subject group demonstrated a significantly better outcome than the bilateral CI group. Some top-performing EAS users came very close to the results of normal-hearing listeners.

Turner et al. [39] could not find better SRTs in simulated EAS listening compared to simulated CI stimulation in a continuous noise condition, whereas in a more complex scenario with competitive talkers, better SRTs were found in the EAS group. The results were confirmed in a small sample of EAS users compared to a group of CI users.

In the present study, the noise in the spatially separated noise condition S0N60 was directed towards the better ear. In the conditions in either noise or reverberation, there was a clinically relevant tendency of better SRTs in the bilateral groups (either EAS or CI) compared to the bimodal CI/EAS groups. For all EAS/CI subject groups, pairwise comparisons revealed a significantly lower monosyllable recognition score in the worse ear. However, this difference was larger in the bimodal CI (28.5%) and EAS (36.4%) groups than in the bilateral CI (12.2%) and EAS (15.8%) groups.

The mean age of the groups with bimodal or bilateral CI stimulation was almost 10 years lower than in the respective EAS groups. It is known that speech perception scores in noise decrease with increasing age, even in normal hearing subjects and when partialling out a potential age-related hearing loss [40]. Furthermore, a recent study reported that age is the only predictive factor for speech perception performance in noise in CI subjects [41]. Therefore, the EAS effect found in previous studies was probably absent in the present study because the age of the CI subject groups was lower. However, testing age-matched subject groups is oftentimes hard to realise in studies with EAS subjects since this is a rather rare subject population.

It has to be noted that in the spatially separated speech in the noise condition, the best performing subject showing SRTs and SRM closest to the NH subjects was in the bilateral EAS group with exceptionally good residual hearing in both ears (subject EAS_BL6 in Table 4).

4.4. Limitation of the Study

The presented work is not without limitations. As the group of EAS users is generally a small population, the number of cases tested in this study is correspondingly low. Studies with larger case numbers would be desirable, so that a stronger correlation between residual hearing and hearing performance in the reverberation could possibly be shown. This was also the reason why it was not possible to match the age of the different study groups (see previous section). Furthermore, the test in the spatially separated condition was always conducted presenting the noise on the EAS ear. Further experiments with the presentation of noise in the contralateral ear were of interest, as SRM would probably be higher in such a test condition.

5. Conclusions

The test procedure, which employed loudspeaker-based room simulation, revealed that reverberation has a detrimental impact on SRT across all subject groups. Only NH subjects achieved spatial release from masking in reverberation, whereas no beneficial effect of spatial separation of speech and noise was found in any CI/EAS group, when noise was presented towards the better hearing ear.

No beneficial effect of combined electric–acoustic stimulation compared to electric stimulation on speech perception in reverberation was found. Further studies on this research question using age-matched subject groups are desirable.

Author Contributions: Conceptualisation, T.W. and U.B.; methodology, T.W.; software, T.W.; validation, T.W., C.K. and U.B.; formal analysis, C.K. and T.W.; investigation, C.K.; resources, U.B. and T.S.; data curation, C.K. and T.W.; writing—original draft preparation, C.K.; writing—review and editing, C.K., T.W., U.B. and T.S.; visualisation, C.K. and T.W.; supervision, T.W.; project administration, T.W. and U.B. All authors have read and agreed to the published version of the manuscript.

Funding: This research received no external funding.

Institutional Review Board Statement: The study was conducted in accordance with the Declaration of Helsinki, and approved by the Institutional Ethics Committee University Hospital Frankfurt (application number: 164/16, 29 June 2016).

Informed Consent Statement: Informed consent was obtained from all subjects involved in the study.

Data Availability Statement: The raw data supporting the conclusions of this article will be made available by the authors on request.

Acknowledgments: The authors would like to thank the Moessner Foundation Frankfurt. Some of the hardware used in the study was sponsored by the foundation.

Conflicts of Interest: The authors declare no conflicts of interest.

References

1. Gifford, R.H.; Loiselle, L.; Natale, S.; Sheffield, S.W.; Sunderhaus, L.W.; S Dietrich, M.; Dorman, M.F. Speech Under-standing in Noise for Adults with Cochlear Implants: Effects of Hearing Configuration, Source Location Certainty, and Head Movement. *J. Speech Lang. Hear. Res.* **2018**, *61*, 1306–1321. [CrossRef] [PubMed]
2. Poissant, S.F.; Whitmal, N.A.; Freyman, R.L. Effects of reverberation and masking on speech intelligibility in cochlear implant simulations. *J. Acoust. Soc. Am.* **2006**, *119*, 1606–1615. [CrossRef] [PubMed]
3. Whitmal, N.A.; Poissant, S.F. Effects of source-to-listener distance and masking on perception of cochlear implant processed speech in reverberant rooms. *J. Acoust. Soc. Am.* **2009**, *126*, 2556–2569. [CrossRef]
4. Misurelli, S.M.; Litovsky, R.Y. Spatial release from masking in children with bilateral cochlear implants and with normal hearing: Effect of target-interferer similarity. *J. Acoust. Soc. Am.* **2015**, *138*, 319–331. [CrossRef]
5. Litovsky, R.Y. Spatial Release from Masking. *Acoust. Today* **2012**, *8*, 18–25. [CrossRef]
6. Gifford, R.H.; Dorman, M.F.; Sheffield, S.W.; Teece, K.; Olund, A.P. Availability of binaural cues for bilateral implant recipients and bimodal listeners with and without preserved hearing in the implanted ear. *Audiol. Neurootol.* **2014**, *19*, 57–71. [CrossRef] [PubMed]
7. Williges, B.; Dietz, M.; Hohmann, V.; Jürgens, T. Spatial Release From Masking in Simulated Cochlear Implant Users With and Without Access to Low-Frequency Acoustic Hearing. *Trends Hear.* **2015**, *19*, 2331216515616940. [CrossRef] [PubMed]
8. Kokkinakis, K.; Loizou, P.C. The impact of reverberant self-masking and overlap-masking effects on speech intelligibility by cochlear implant listeners (L). *J. Acoust. Soc. Am.* **2011**, *130*, 1099–1102. [CrossRef]
9. Mühler, R.; Ziese, M.; Rostalski, D.; Verhey, J.L. Zur Wahrnehmung verhallter Sprache mit Cochleaimplantaten. [On the perception of reverberated speech with cochlear implants]. *HNO* **2014**, *1*, 35–40. [CrossRef]
10. Desmond, J.M.; Collins, L.M.; Throckmorton, C.S. The effects of reverberant self- and overlap-masking on speech recognition in cochlear implant listeners. *J. Acoust. Soc. Am.* **2014**, *135*, EL304–EL310. [CrossRef]
11. Eichenauer, A.; Baumann, U.; Stöver, T.; Weißgerber, T. Interleaved Acoustic Environments: Impact of an Auditory Scene Classification Procedure on Speech Perception in Cochlear Implant Users. *Trends Hear.* **2021**, *25*, 23312165211014118. [CrossRef]
12. Kressner, A.A.; Westermann, A.; Buchholz, J.M. The impact of reverberation on speech intelligibility in cochlear implant recipients. *J. Acoust. Soc. Am.* **2018**, *144*, 1113. [CrossRef] [PubMed]
13. Hazrati, O.; Lee, J.; Loizou, P.C. Blind binary masking for reverberation suppression in cochlear implants. *J. Acoust. Soc. Am.* **2013**, *133*, 1607–1614. [CrossRef] [PubMed]
14. Hu, Y.; Kokkinakis, K. Effects of early and late reflections on intelligibility of reverberated speech by cochlear im-plant listeners. *J. Acoust. Soc. Am.* **2014**, *135*, EL22–EL28. [CrossRef]
15. Hazrati, O.; Loizou, P.C. The combined effects of reverberation and noise on speech intelligibility by cochlear implant listeners. *Int. J. Audiol.* **2012**, *51*, 437–443. [CrossRef]
16. Darwin, C.J.; Hukin, R.W. Effectiveness of spatial cues, prosody, and talker characteristics in selective attention. *J. Acoust. Soc. Am.* **2000**, *107*, 970–977. [CrossRef]
17. Helms Tillery, K.; Brown, C.A.; Bacon, S.P. Comparing the effects of reverberation and of noise on speech recognition in simulated electric-acoustic listening. *J. Acoust. Soc. Am.* **2012**, *131*, 416–423. [CrossRef] [PubMed]
18. Badajoz-Davila, J.; Buchholz, J.M.; Van-Hoesel, R. Effect of noise and reverberation on speech intelligibility for cochlear implant recipients in realistic sound environments. *J. Acoust. Soc. Am.* **2020**, *147*, 3538–3549. [CrossRef] [PubMed]
19. Von Ilberg, C.; Baumann, U.; Kiefer, J.; Tillein, J.; Adunka, O.F. Electric-acoustic stimulation of the auditory system: A review of the first decade. *Audiol. Neurootol.* **2011**, *16* (Suppl. S2), 1–30. [CrossRef]
20. Lorens, A.; Polak, M.; Piotrowska, A.; Skarzynski, H. Outcomes of treatment of partial deafness with cochlear implantation: A DUET study. *Laryngoscope* **2008**, *118*, 288–294. [CrossRef]
21. Helbig, S.; Baumann, U.; Helbig, M.; von Malsen-Waldkirch, N.; Gstoettner, W. A new combined speech processor for electric and acoustic stimulation--eight months experience. *ORL J. Oto-Rhino-Lary* **2008**, *70*, 359–365. [CrossRef]
22. Weißgerber, T.; Stöver, T.; Baumann, U. Speech perception in noise: Impact of directional microphones in users of combined electric-acoustic stimulation. *PLoS ONE* **2019**, *14*, e0213251. [CrossRef] [PubMed]
23. Dorman, M.F.; Gifford, R.H. Combining acoustic and electric stimulation in the service of speech recognition. *Int. J. Audiol.* **2010**, *49*, 912–919. [CrossRef]
24. Dunn, C.C.; Perreau, A.; Gantz, B.; Tyler, R.S. Benefits of localization and speech perception with multiple noise sources in listeners with a short-electrode cochlear implant. *J. Am. Acad. Audiol.* **2010**, *21*, 44–51. [CrossRef] [PubMed]
25. Rader, T.; Fastl, H.; Baumann, U. Speech perception with combined electric-acoustic stimulation and bilateral cochlear implants in a multisource noise field. *Ear Hear.* **2013**, *34*, 324–332. [CrossRef]

26. Gifford, R.H.; Dorman, M.F.; Skarzynski, H.; Lorens, A.; Polak, M.; Driscoll, C.L.; Roland, P.; Buchman, C.A. Cochlear implantation with hearing preservation yields significant benefit for speech recognition in complex listening environments. *Ear Hear.* **2013**, *34*, 413–425. [CrossRef] [PubMed]
27. Dorman, M.F.; Spahr, A.J.; Loiselle, L.; Zhang, T.; Cook, S.; Brown, C.; Yost, W. Localization and speech understanding by a patient with bilateral cochlear implants and bilateral hearing preservation. *Ear Hear.* **2013**, *34*, 245–248. [CrossRef]
28. Zhang, T.; Dorman, M.F.; Spahr, A.J. Information From the Voice Fundamental Frequency (F0) Region Accounts for the Majority of the Benefit When Acoustic Stimulation Is Added to Electric Stimulation. *Ear Hear.* **2010**, *31*, 63–69. [CrossRef]
29. Fu, Q.-J.; Shannon, R.V.; Wang, X. Effects of noise and spectral resolution on vowel and consonant recognition: Acoustic and electric hearing. *J. Acoust. Soc. Am.* **1998**, *104*, 3586–3596. [CrossRef]
30. Hahlbrock, K.-H. Über Sprachaudiometrie und neue Wörterteste. [Speech audiometry and new word-tests]. *Archiv. Ohren-Nasen-Kehlkopfheilkd.* **1953**, *162*, 394–431. [CrossRef]
31. Weißgerber, T.; Rader, T.; Baumann, U. Impact of a moving noise masker on speech perception in cochlear implant users. *PLoS ONE* **2015**, *10*, e0126133. [CrossRef] [PubMed]
32. Eichenauer, A.; Baumann, U.; Weißgerber, T. Implementierung und Evaluation einer akustischen Raumsimulation für audiologische Testungen. [Implementation and evaluation of acoustic room simulation for audiological testing]. *GMS Z. Audiol.—Audiol. Acoust.* **2020**, *2*, Doc06. [CrossRef]
33. Wagener, K.; Brand, T.; Kollmeier, B. Entwicklung und Evaluation eines Satztests für die deutsche Sprache. Teil II: Optimierung des Oldenburger Satztests. [Development and evaluation of a German sentence test. Part II: Optimization of the Oldenburg sentence test]. *Z. Audiol.* **1999**, *38*, 44–56.
34. Kokkinakis, K.; Hazrati, O.; Loizou, P.C. A channel-selection criterion for suppressing reverberation in cochlear implants. *J. Acoust. Soc. Am.* **2011**, *129*, 3221–3232. [CrossRef] [PubMed]
35. Rennies, J.; Kidd, G. Benefit of binaural listening as revealed by speech intelligibility and listening effort. *J. Acoust. Soc. Am.* **2018**, *144*, 2147. [CrossRef]
36. Weißgerber, T.; Rader, T.; Baumann, U. Effectiveness of Directional Microphones in Bilateral/Bimodal Cochlear Implant Users-Impact of Spatial and Temporal Noise Characteristics. *Otol. Neurotol.* **2017**, *38*, e551–e557. [CrossRef]
37. Gantz, B.J.; Turner, C.W. Combining acoustic and electrical hearing. *Laryngoscope* **2003**, *113*, 1726–1730. [CrossRef]
38. Büchner, A.; Schüssler, M.; Battmer, R.D.; Stöver, T.; Lesinski-Schiedat, A.; Lenarz, T. Impact of Low-Frequency Hearing. *Audiol. Neurootol.* **2009**, *14*, 8–13. [CrossRef]
39. Turner, C.W.; Gantz, B.J.; Vidal, C.; Behrens, A.; Henry, B.A. Speech recognition in noise for cochlear implant listeners: Benefits of residual acoustic hearing. *J. Acoust. Soc. Am.* **2004**, *115*, 1729. [CrossRef]
40. Weißgerber, T.; Müller, C.; Stöver, T.; Baumann, U. Age Differences in Speech Perception in Noise and Sound Localization in Individuals with Subjective Normal Hearing. *Front. Psychol.* **2022**, *13*, 845285. [CrossRef]
41. Weissgerber, T.; Löschner, M.; Stöver, T.; Baumann, U. Outcome Prediction of Speech Perception in Quiet and in Noise for Cochlear Implant Candidates Based on Pre-Operative Measures. *J. Clin. Med.* **2024**, *13*, 994. [CrossRef] [PubMed]

Journal of
Clinical Medicine

MDPI

Article

Enhancing Cochlear Implant Outcomes across Age Groups: The Interplay of Forward Focus and Advanced Combination Encoder Coding Strategies in Noisy Conditions

Telse M. Wagner *, Luise Wagner, Stefan K. Plontke and Torsten Rahne

Department of Otorhinolaryngology, University Medicine Halle, Ernst-Grube-Straße 40, 06120 Halle (Saale), Germany; luise.wagner@uk-halle.de (L.W.); stefan.plontke@uk-halle.de (S.K.P.); torsten.rahne@uk-halle.de (T.R.)
* Correspondence: telse.wagner@student.uni-halle.de

Abstract: Background: Hearing in noise is challenging for cochlear implant users and requires significant listening effort. This study investigated the influence of ForwardFocus and number of maxima of the Advanced Combination Encoder (ACE) strategy, as well as age, on speech recognition threshold and listening effort in noise. **Methods:** A total of 33 cochlear implant recipients were included (age $\leq$ 40 years: n = 15, >40 years: n = 18). The Oldenburg Sentence Test was used to measure 50% speech recognition thresholds (SRT50) in fluctuating and stationary noise. Speech was presented frontally, while three frontal or rear noise sources were used, and the number of ACE maxima varied between 8 and 12. **Results:** ForwardFocus significantly improved the SRT50 when noise was presented from the back, independent of subject age. The use of 12 maxima further improved the SRT50 when ForwardFocus was activated and when noise and speech were presented frontally. Listening effort was significantly worse in the older age group compared to the younger age group and was reduced by ForwardFocus but not by increasing the number of ACE maxima. **Conclusion:** Forward Focus can improve speech recognition in noisy environments and reduce listening effort, especially in older cochlear implant users.

Keywords: age-related hearing loss; cochlear implant; ForwardFocus; hearing effort; hearing in noise; speech recognition

1. Introduction

Hearing is one of the most essential prerequisites for communication [1] and an important component of social interaction and quality of life [2,3]. Untreated hearing disorders can impair cognitive performance and even contribute to the development of dementia [4–6]. If conventional hearing aid treatment is insufficient or not indicated, cochlear implants (CIs) may be an alternative to facilitate hearing by bypassing the inner ear and stimulating the auditory nerve electrically [7]. CI-mediated hearing differs from normal hearing in quality and timbre [8] and also speech perception is still not comparable to normal hearing.

Besides speech recognition in quiet [9], cochlear implantation also aims for good speech recognition in noise [10–12]. Hey et al. [13], however, showed that CI users with high levels of open-set speech recognition in quiet may still have poor hearing in noise compared to normal-hearing listeners [14]. To overcome this deficit, noise reduction algorithms were developed to improve the signal-to-noise ratio (SNR) and thus hearing with a CI [15]. The benefit of noise reduction technologies was, however, reduced with a reduction in the number of competing speakers [14,16,17]. A typical situation is the so-called cocktail party setting [18]. Normal hearing listeners can focus their listening attention on one specific speaker, even if there are other conversations in their immediate surroundings. In contrast, CI users need special noise reduction technologies to focus on the speaking person. Wimmer et al. [19] showed that in those situations speech recognition and SNR can be improved by using directional microphones.

A relatively new CI sound-processing algorithm is ForwardFocus (FF). ForwardFocus attenuates sounds from behind while preserving sounds from the front, in order to increase speech recognition in noise by increasing the SNR. To help CI users in focusing on frontal speakers more than directional microphones can do, FF was first implemented in the audio processor of the Nucleus 7 system (Cochlear, Sydney, Australia) [14].

Hey et al. [14] showed a superiority of 5.8 dB SNR with FF in comparison to directional microphone technology if the noise was presented from behind (90°, 180° and 270°). The impact of FF on speech perception in frontal noise presentation has not been investigated in detail. Since fluctuating noise signals are considered to have high ecological validity [20,21], an effect of FF on speech perception in icra5, a noise signal developed for audiological testing resembling the sound of a single speaker with pauses of 250 ms [22], would be expected as well.

Another option to increase speech recognition in Nucleus CI users is the Advanced Combination Encoder (ACE) strategy, which selects only the channels with the highest spectral energy in each stimulation cycle (number of maxima). It has been shown that the ACE algorithm is sensitive to noise since the wrong maxima could be selected, especially in speech gaps [23]. Berg et al. [24], however, showed that the maxima selection strategy of ACE improved sentences in noise discrimination and spectral modulation detection compared to a 16-channel continuously interleaved samples (CIS) strategy. Using sixteen versus eight maxima led to a significantly better understanding of monosyllables and sentences in a 20-talker babble noise signal for presenting speech and noise from the front (S_0N_0).

While a decrease in hearing in general underlies a degradation of peripheral hearing and cognitive decline, it is still unclear how age affects hearing with CIs. So far, only a few studies have examined aging in CI users and no study has investigated aging effects for FF and ACE maxima conditions. Shew et al. [25] examined two groups of bimodal CI users aged below and above 65 years. No difference between the age groups was found when hearing in quiet was measured, but the addition of noise resulted in a disproportional decline for the older participants. As a possible explanation, Füllgrabe [26] found that temporal processing deteriorates with age, starting in early midlife. The first significant deficits were observed in normal-hearing participants between the ages of 40 and 49 years, even in the absence of peripheral hearing loss. Above the age of 40 years, the maximum word recognition score also starts to decline, as observed in a large cohort [27].

Since CI outcome depends on cognitive factors, listening effort, as measurement of these factors, has been introduced as an important assessment [28]. After cochlear implantation, the available acoustic and spectro-temporal cues are limited, which would cause an increased listening effort [9]. This assumption was recently confirmed by a review of 24 studies that showed higher levels of listening effort in CI users when compared to normal-hearing controls using scales, questionnaires, and electroencephalogram measurements [29]. Nevertheless, the main factors leading to this difference still need to be clarified. It is hypothesized that the technical parameters of cochlear implants greatly impact listening effort, more than age or cognitive factors do [9]. Other studies discussed the effects of cognitive factors such as working memory capacity or inhibitory control on listening effort [29,30] and found effects of aging on listening effort in CI users [31]. According to a study by Perrau et al., other variables, such as the duration of CI use and the age of onset of hearing loss, were not significantly related to listening effort [31].

This study aimed to evaluate the effects of FF and number of ACE maxima on speech recognition and listening effort in spatial conditions when fluctuating noise is presented from the front or the back. A younger group and an older group of CI users were included and compared to age-matched reference data of normal-hearing listeners [32]. We hypothesized that an increased number of ACE maxima would increase the spectral information of the CIs and therefore could reduce listening effort in noise and that the increased SNR by using FF would reduce listening effort in noise as well.

2. Materials and Methods

In a prospective, non-interventional exploratory cohort study, CI users between 18 and 80 years of age were included and allocated to the age groups of $\leq$40 years and >40 years. Inclusion criteria were a post-lingually acquired CI indication; use of a Nucleus CI24RE, CI5xx, or CI6xx device (Cochlear, Sydney, Australia) with at least 20 active electrode contacts; use of the ACE coding strategy for at least six months; being a German native speaker; and having a CI-aided monosyllabic word recognition score (WRS) in quiet of at least 50% at 65 dB SPL. This study was conducted in a laboratory of experimental audiology at a university hearing and implant center. This study was approved by the local ethical review board (approval number 2021-044) and conducted in compliance with the Declaration of Helsinki. Informed written consent was obtained from all participants.

All measurements were performed in a unilateral setting with the same Nucleus 7 audio processor. For bilaterally implanted CI users, the side with the better WRS was chosen. Each individual patient's device fitting was used as base for the study settings: eight maxima without FF (M8/FF−), eight maxima with activated FF (M8/FF+), and twelve maxima with activated FF (M12/FF+). If the individual setting did not allow for twelve maxima, the largest possible number of maxima was used instead.

Participants were positioned in a circle at a distance of 1 m from the loudspeakers in a sound-attenuated room. The head was fixed with a papillon head fixation system. The German matrix sentence test OLSA (HörTech, Oldenburg, Germany) [9,33,34] was utilized to measure the 50% speech recognition threshold (SRT_{50}) in noise with a constant sound pressure level of 65 dB. Figure 1 shows the three spatial configurations of speech and noise presentation. The speech signal (S) of the target speaker was always presented in front (0°, S_0). Noise signals (N) were either the generic noise of the OLSA with a male voice (olnoise) or the icra5 fluctuating noise of the OLSA. In the frontal noise condition, the noise signals were presented from 0°, +45°, and −45° (S_0N_{front}). The rear noise presentation locations were 180°, +135°, and −135° (S_0N_{rear}). The S_0N_0 condition was used as the reference and training condition. Participants were presented with lists of 20 sentences with adaptive speech levels in continuous noise. Within the adaptive measurement of SRT_{50}, after every sentence, the sound pressure level was adjusted based on the participant's response to the preceding sentence. Two training lists, one for olnoise and one for icra5, were used before the 12 test runs started in a pseudorandom sequence. For the spatial conditions of S_0N_{front} and S_0N_{rear}, the test runs comprised olnoise with M8/FF− and icra5 with M8/FF−, M8/FF+, and M12/FF+.

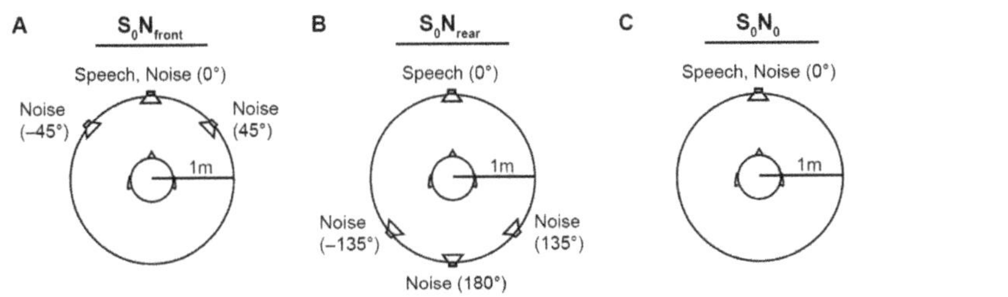

Figure 1. Experimental conditions with speech presented from the front (0°): (**A**) frontal noise condition with noise signals presented from 0°, +45°, and −45° (S_0N_{front}); (**B**) rear noise condition with noise signals presented from 180°, +135°, and −135° (S_0N_{rear}); and (**C**) S_0N_0 reference condition with only one frontal noise source (0°).

Listening effort was measured using the "Adaptive Categorical Listening Effort Scaling" (ACALES) test (Hörtech, Oldenburg, Germany) [9,35,36] in the S_0N_0 condition. The participants were asked to rate their listening effort on a scale of eight response categories ranging from 'no effort' to 'only noise' following the frontal presentation of two sentences from the OLSA test in 65 dB SPL icra5 noise. Based on the previous rating, the SNR was changed adaptively for every set of two sentences. SNR limits of −40 dB and +20 dB were applied. The SNR_{cut}, which is the SNR at which a moderate effort (4 effort scale categorical units, ESCUs) was measured, was assessed for all experimental conditions.

The SRT_{50} and SNR_{cut} distributions were descriptively reported and analyzed. Normality was assessed through the Shapiro–Wilk test. To compare the distributions of SRT_{50} between the spatial configurations, the signal processing settings, and age, an ANOVA for repeated measures with the within-subject factors of 'spatial condition', 'FF', and 'Maxima' and the between-subject factor of 'age group' was used. Mauchly's test was utilized to verify the assumption of sphericity and Greenhouse–Geisser correction was applied if necessary. The effect of the age group on the SNR_{cut} was analyzed with an ANOVA for all used experimental conditions. Bonferroni correction was applied to adjust the degrees of freedom for all post hoc comparisons. The required sample size was based on the SRT_{50} as the primary endpoint with an assumed standard deviation of 2 dB. To calculate the 95% confidence intervals with an assumed length of 2 dB, a sample size of 18 participants per age group resulted. This is comparable to studies that have already been successfully conducted with similar methodologies and research questions. The statistical analyses were performed using version 28 of the SPSS software from IBM in Ehningen, Germany. The level of significance was set to $p = 0.05$.

3. Results

Thirty-three participants were recruited. One participant with SRT_{50} values above 30 dB SNR was excluded from the analysis. Table 1 provides the demographic and implantation data of all analyzed participants. Electrode insertion was mostly through the round window, in four cases after a partial or subtotal cochleoectomy, and in two cases through a cochlestomy.

Table 1. Anamnestic data and baseline characteristics.

	Age Groups		
Characteristics	**≤40 Years**	**>40 Years**	**All**
Number	14	18	32
Age, mean (SD), years	28.6 (7.9)	70.0 (7.2)	51.9 (22.1)
Median [25th, 75th percentiles]	27.0 [20.0, 36.3]	69.5 [62.8, 76.3]	61.0 [29.5, 71.5]
Men/women, N	9/5	13/5	22/10
Right/left CI, N	5/9	8/10	13/19
Word recognition, mean (SD), % correct at 65 dB SPL			
Ipsilateral	71 (17)	73 (15)	72 (15)
Median [25th, 75th percentiles]	73 [58, 85]	75 [60, 85]	75 [60, 85]
Contralateral	65 (40)	59 (23)	62 (31)
Median [25th, 75th percentiles]	78 [34, 100]	65 [53, 75]	68 [48, 84]
Active electrodes, mean (SD), *n*	21.8 (0.8)	21.8 (0.5)	21.8 (0.6)
Median [25th, 75th percentiles]	22.0 [22.0, 22.0]	22.0 [22.0, 22.0]	22.0 [22.0, 22.0]
Pulse width, mean (SD), ms	35.5 (13.7)	29.7 (7.5)	32.3 (10.9)
Median [25th, 75th percentiles]	37.0 [25.0, 37.0]	25.0 [25.0, 37.0]	25.0 [25.0, 37.0]
Stimulation rate, mean (SD), Hz	921.4 (80.2)	977.8 (186.5)	953.1 (150.2)
Median [25th, 75th percentiles]	900.0 [900.0, 900.0]	900.0 [900.0, 1200.0]	900.0 [900.0, 900.0]
CI usage per day, mean (SD), hours	11.5 (5.5)	13.7 (2.3)	12.8 (4.1)
Median [25th, 75th percentiles]	13.0 [8.8, 15.3]	14.0 [12.0, 15.2]	14.0 [11.3, 15.0]
CI experience, mean (SD), years	5.9 (4.9)	5.1 (3.2)	5.4 (4.0)
Median [25th, 75th percentiles]	4.5 [1.7, 9.5]	4.0 [2.8, 7.0]	4.0 [2.0, 9.0]

Figure 2 shows the SRT_{50} for all spatial and noise conditions for the two age groups. The respective mean SRT_{50} and standard deviations are shown in Table 2. The ANOVA of SRT_{50} shows no effect of the age group ($F(1,30) = 2.3$; $p = 0.142$). The effects of spatial condition ($F(1.5,45.3) = 35.5$; $p < 0.001$), noise ($F(1,30) = 7.6$; $p = 0.010$), and the interaction of spatial condition and noise ($F(1.5,45.5) = 11.7$; $p < 0.001$) were significant. Post hoc comparisons show better SRT_{50} for olnoise (−4.53 dB SNR) as compared to icra5 (−2.45 dB SNR). The SRT_{50} for S_0N_{rear} (−5.69 dB SNR) was significantly better than for S_0N_0 (−2.63 dB SNR), all other differences were not significant. Since age group had no effect on the SRT_{50} results, both groups were combined for further analysis.

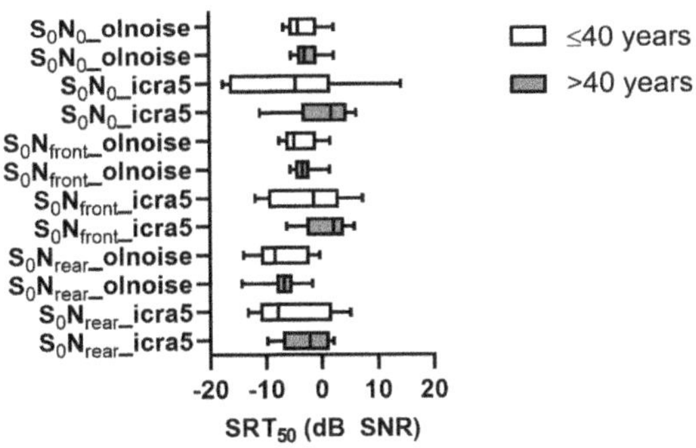

Figure 2. Speech recognition threshold (SRT_{50}) for all spatial and noise conditions for the two age groups, ≤40 years (white) and >40 years (grey), presented as boxplots for all analyzed participants with deactivated FF and using 8 ACE maxima (M8/FF−). The whiskers show minimum and maximum values.

Table 2. Speech recognition and listening effort in noise outcomes.

Age Group, Years		**Age Group, Years**		
Outcome		**≤40**	**>40**	**Total**
Speech recognition in noise SRT_{50} in dB SNR, mean (SD)				
olnoise M8/FF−	S_0N_0	−3.2 (2.9)	−2.3 (2.4)	−2.7 (2.6)
	S_0N_{front}	−3.9 (3.0)	−3.1 (1.9)	−3.5 (2.4)
	S_0N_{rear}	−7.5 (4.4)	−7.0 (2.8)	−7.2 (3.5)
icra5 M8/FF−	S_0N_0	−5.1 (10.6)	0.1 (5.1)	−2.2 (8.2)
	S_0N_{front}	−2.6 (7.1)	1.0 (3.8)	−0.6 (5.7)
	S_0N_{rear}	−5.3 (6.8)	−2.9 (4.1)	−4.0 (5.5)
icra5 M8/FF+	S_0N_0	−4.7 (9.9)	0.7 (5.5)	−1.6 (8.1)
	S_0N_{front}	−2.8 (6.6)	1.0 (3.7)	−0.7 (5.4)
	S_0N_{rear}	−9.7 (4.0)	−8.7 (2.9)	−9.1 (3.4)
icra5 M12/FF+	S_0N_0	−5.9 (8.8)	−0.2 (5.0)	−2.7 (7.4)
	S_0N_{front}	−3.1 (6.6)	0.5 (4.1)	−1.1 (5.5)
	S_0N_{rear}	−10.3 (4.6)	−9.5 (2.4)	−9.8 (3.5)
Listening effort in noise SNR_{cut} in dB SNR (SD)				
icra5 M8/FF−	S_0N_0	−4.8 (7.8)	4.7 (5.7)	0.1 (8.2)
icra5 M8/FF+	S_0N_0	−4.3 (7.4)	2.3 (4.8)	−0.9 (6.9)
icra5 M12/FF+	S_0N_0	−3.7 (7.0)	3.5 (5.4)	0.1 (7.1)

Abbreviations: SNR: signal-to-noise ratio; SD: standard deviation; SPL: sound pressure level; SRT50: 50% speech reception threshold; SNR_{cut}: signal-to-noise ratio at moderate listening effort.

The effect of FF on the SRT_{50} is shown in Figure 3, together with reference data of normal-hearing listeners [32]. FF improved the SRT_{50} in the S_0N_{rear} condition from −4.0 dB SNR (SD: 5.5) to −9.1 dB SNR (SD: 3.4) ($p < 0.001$), but not in the other spatial conditions.

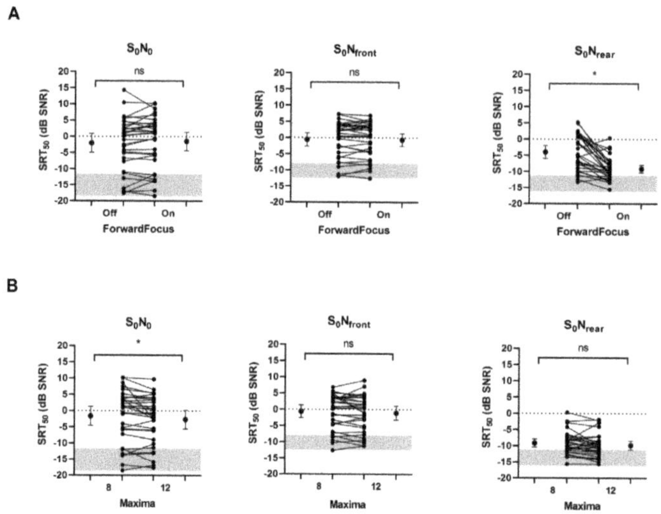

Figure 3. (**A**) Effect of ForwardFocus and (**B**) number of ACE maxima on the speech recognition threshold in noise (SRT_{50}) for different spatial conditions of signal and noise presentations. Individual data are presented together with the means ± SD. Significant differences are marked with an asterisk ($p < 0.05$); ns: not significant. The reference data for normal hearing listeners [32] are displayed as grey bars (means ± SD).

The effect of an increased number of ACE maxima is also shown in Figure 3. The missing values of two participants were imputed based on the respective mean SRT_{50} of the age group (S_0N_0: −2.69 dB, S_0N_{front}: −1.09 dB, S_0N_{rear}: −9.81 dB). The increased number of ACE maxima improved the SRT_{50} in the S_0N_0 condition from −1.6 dB SNR (SD: 8.1) to −2.7 dB SNR (SD: 7.4) ($p = 0.033$), but not in the other spatial conditions.

All participants participated in the ACALES test. The test was terminated if the SNR of the stimulus presentation exceeded 16 dB. This affected four participants in the younger age group and six participants in the older age group. In addition, five more participants in the older age group could not complete the test for only one or two of the three conditions. In these cases, the missing values were replaced by a value of 10 dB SNR.

Figure 4 shows the SNR_{cut} results of the ACALES test for listening effort. The mean values are reported in Table 2. The ANOVA of SNR_{cut} shows an effect of age group in the M8/FF− condition ($F(1,21) = 11.5$; $p = 0.003$), the M8/FF+ condition ($F(1,21) = 6.7$; $p = 0.017$), and the M12/FF+ condition ($F(1,21) = 7.6$; $p = 0.012$). In the older age group, SNRcut showed a significant increase of 9.5 dB for M8/FF−, 6.6 dB for M8/FF+, and 7.2 dB for M12/FF+. In the younger group, no significant differences in SNR_{cut} were measured between the FF and ACE maxima conditions. FF significantly improved the SNR_{cut} by 2.4 dB ($p = 0.027$) in the older age group; however, the additional increase in ACE maxima worsened it by 1.2 dB ($p = 0.0495$).

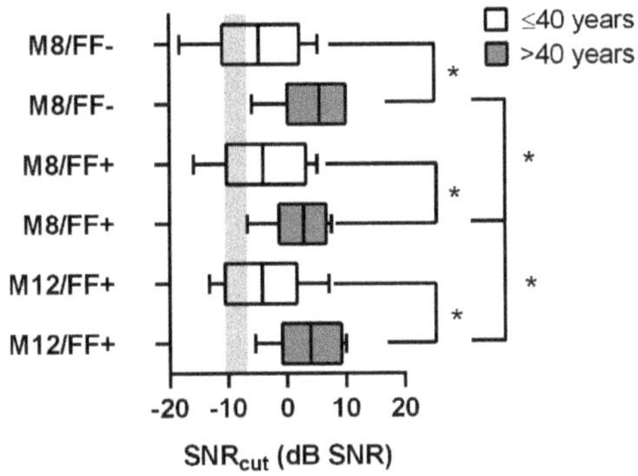

Figure 4. Listening effort in noise displayed as boxplots for different signal processing conditions and age groups. Significant differences are marked with an asterisk ($p < 0.05$). The reference data for normal hearing listeners [32] are displayed as grey bars (means ± SD).

4. Discussion

The results show that FF improves speech recognition in noise when fluctuating noise is presented from rear directions and has no effect on SRT if noise is frontally presented. Since noise sources from behind often occur in daily life, this result is relevant for CI users. However, not all CI users benefited from activated FF, and 4 of the 32 analyzed participants even achieved worse results. Possible reasons for this are that two of these four participants reported very short daily CI wearing times (1 h/d) and were potentially not used to hearing with the CI in general. For another participant, we suspect that cognitive factors interacted with performance in our study.

Apparently, there is a slight trend that participants with poor speech recognition in noise profited more from FF than participants with good speech recognition in noise. An analysis of two previous studies [14,37] indicates similar characteristics in the corresponding patient cohorts. However, this needs to be confirmed in a dedicated future investigation. Overall, the FF-induced improvement in speech recognition in noise for the S_0N_{rear} condition is in line with the results of Hey et al. for the $S_0N_{90,180,270}$ condition [14]. The present study complements those findings by showing similar results with the Nucleus 7 audio processor. As expected from the signal processing design of FF [14], speech recognition in noise could not be improved if noise came from the front (S_0N_{front}, S_0N_0).

A limitation of this unilateral study design is that in bilaterally implanted CI users, FF was only activated in one CI. Those participants reported a somehow unbalanced hearing and would potentially benefit even more from FF being activated in both audio processors. Also, the duration of deafness before CI implantation and CI experience could influence speech recognition in noise. To avoid a resulting bias, both age groups were balanced according to CI experience.

When the number of ACE maxima was increased to 12, the results show significant SRT_{50} improvements only for the S_0N_0 condition. We hypothesize that in less complex listening situations, such as the S_0N_0 condition, spatial cues cannot be utilized to separate speech and noise. An increased number of maxima would then potentially provide more speech-related information, which helps to better discriminate speech from noise. If noise comes from three directions (S_0N_{front} or S_0N_{rear}) and speech only from one, ACE maxima selection would also pick up signals from all three directions based on their amplitudes and increase the difficulty of discriminating the speech signal from noise based on spatial information alone.

These results are in line with those of Berg et al. [24], who showed significant improvements using 16 versus 8 maxima in the ACE strategy for sentence recognition in noise. The S_0N_0 condition is suitable for standardized audiometry but with questionable impact for everyday hearing. We assume that FF and increased ACE maxima could be used simultaneously to achieve better speech recognition in such less-complex situations. Nevertheless, for difficult listening conditions (S_0N_{rear}), which often appear in real-life settings, the results show that increasing the number of maxima from 8 to 12 does not provide significant benefits over FF in speech perception overall. In the present study, however, some participants could only be measured with 9 to 11 maxima instead of 12, and other parameters such as electrode-to-modiolus distance depending on the type of electrode carrier used also varied between participants. We recommend future studies to investigate the number of ACE maxima independently of FF in different spatial conditions. Also, in our data, we could see some that patients improved their results and could observe a trend that the best mean value for speech perception (−9.8 dB), whenever not significant, was found in the S_0N_{rear} condition using 12 maxima.

In our study, age group did not affect speech recognition thresholds in noise. In contrast to a study by Füllgrabe et al. [26], which described a decreased processing of temporal fine structure cues with age, starting between 40 and 49 years, even without peripheral hearing loss in normal hearing listeners, we did not find a deterioration in SRT_{50} in fluctuating noise with age. Also contrasting with our results, Shew et al. [25] demonstrated that the addition of noise disproportionally affects the speech recognition of adults over 65 years old. Either age did not have a significant impact in our test setting at all or the detrimental effect of age has a later onset than reflected in our age groups, which had a cutoff at 40 years, or even neither is true. The time of implantation and daily wearing time likely affect hearing in CI users more than age does [38,39].

Compared with age-specific reference data for the same spatial signal and noise configurations [32], the present results demonstrate that some CI users are able to perform similar to normal-hearing listeners. Thus, despite the fact that studies often overestimate the performance of CIs due to the experimental design [40,41], we conclude that FF provides a tool that significantly reduces hearing deficits in some situations.

Compared to olnoise, the results show poorer SRT_{50} for fluctuating icra5 noise. This confirms that fluctuating competing signals are more difficult for CI users. [7,14,42] In the same experimental design as in the present study, normal-hearing listeners showed better SRT_{50} in icra5 noise compared to olnoise. While normal-hearing people can benefit from the so-called gap listening [43], CI users could possibly not detect the speech signals in the pauses of only 250 ms within the icra5 noise signal. This is consistent with a study by Rader et al. [44], who were also unable to detect gap listening in CI users in modulated noise.

Although hearing tests in noise are becoming more relevant in everyday clinical practice, their ecological validity needs to be improved [41]. Several studies have shown that fluctuating interfering signals or competing talkers [45] can best reflect everyday situations [42,46]. Hey et al. [41] recently revealed that a stationary noise cannot replace interfering signals if used in speech audiometry. The results of our study are based on the recommended icra5 noise [22,47] and can thus contribute to the standardization of clinical measurements, especially in comparison with the recently published data of normal-hearing subjects [32].

In contrast to the results for speech intelligibility in noise, we found a significant age dependency in listening effort across all experimental conditions. Older CI users (>40 years) showed a larger listening effort in noise than those in the age group $\leq$40 years. Although speech recognition measurements were possible in these participants, some in the group >40 years could not even complete the ACALES test because even the largest possible SNR was rated as too exhausting. This was not observed in the younger age group. The differences between the age groups might result from the deterioration in temporal fine structure processing with age [26] or other cognitive factors like processing speed, executive control, and working memory capacity, which exhibit known age effects [9,30].

We found that FF reduced listening effort only in the group >40 years. From this, we conclude that reducing background noise might reduce cognitive effort and thus listening effort. This finding might be explained by the "Framework for Understanding Effortful Listening" (FUEL) model, which describes listening effort as a multifactorial construct, consisting of cognitive, motivational, and input-related demands. It suggests that speech recognition and listening effort can differ due to individual cognitive factors [9,48]. We assume that the input-related benefits of the FF microphone technology decreased the cognitive demand for speech comprehension, which is considered to be higher in older listeners [49], and led to reduced listening effort in that group. Based on this theory, younger CI users might have more cognitive resources, e.g., better temporal processing, that make listening effort more independent from input-related speech recognition. However, since this study was powered for speech perception in noise, future studies should address the effects of age on listening effort in noise in more detail.

Additionally, FF reduced listening effort for older CI users in the S_0N_0 condition, for which no improvements in speech recognition could be expected. This confirms the theory that speech recognition and listening effort are not aligned, and FF can improve listening effort independently from an improvement in speech recognition.

Another limitation of this study is that some participants were experienced FF users and others activated it for the first time, which could have introduced bias to the results. While data on this subject are very limited, it is being discussed that experienced FF users may have advantages in speech recognition, also in noise, due to training effects comparable to an acclimatization effect of new coding strategies [50].

It was also observed that most CI users had a markedly higher listening effort than normal-hearing listeners, which was reflected in the relatively high dropout rates in the ACALES test. We suggest that future investigations include more spatial conditions, investigating the relation between improved speech recognition scores as for the S_0N_{rear} condition and reduced listening effort, including training with FF to examine this observation more concisely.

Age-mediated cognitive factors or other, not examined, factors linked with auditive processing, such as age at the time of implantation, which can be associated with decreased neuronal plasticity or the time of deafness before implantation, could explain the observed effects of age on listening effort. Our groups, however, were not matched with respect to these factors. Age-dependent listening effort based on cognitive changes should also have affected the normal-hearing reference group of Rahne et al. [32]. However, these data show an age effect only on speech recognition in noise but not on listening effort. This might be explained by the finding of Abdel-Latif and Meister [9] showing that the outcomes of cognitive tests (processing speed, executive control, and working memory capacity) were correlated with age, but no impact of age and cognitive abilities on listening effort in CI users was found. The authors concluded that listening effort was dominated by device-related, technical factors. The results of our study suggest that FF decreases listening effort independently from speech recognition. As a consequence, the assessment of listening effort should be included into clinical routine assessment after CI provision.

To summarize, we conclude that FF can significantly improve speech recognition in the presence of multiple noise sources presented from the rear, which can improve hearing in daily life. ForwardFocus reduced listening effort in older CI users, for whom the listening effort is larger compared to younger and normal-hearing listeners. The number of ACE maxima decreased the speech recognition threshold in noise if speech and noise were frontally presented and did not affect listening effort. Generally, speech recognition in noise was not found to be age-dependent. However, future studies should focus on individual effects of aging and age-related cognitive effects on listening effort in CI users.

Author Contributions: Conceptualization, T.M.W. and T.R.; Methodology, T.M.W. and T.R.; Formal Analysis, T.M.W. and T.R.; Investigation, T.M.W. and L.W.; Resources, T.R. and S.K.P.; Data Curation, T.R.; Writing—Original Draft Preparation, T.M.W. and T.R.; Writing—Review and Editing, T.R., L.W., T.M.W. and S.K.P.; Visualization, T.M.W. and T.R.; Supervision, T.R.; Project Administration, T.R.; Funding Acquisition, T.R. All authors have read and agreed to the published version of the manuscript.

Funding: This research was funded by Cochlear Research and Development Limited, Addlestone, UK, grant number IIR-2317.

Institutional Review Board Statement: The study was conducted in accordance with the Declaration of Helsinki, and the protocol was approved by the Ethics Committee of the Martin Luther University Halle-Wittenberg (21 April 2021; project identification code 2021-044).

Informed Consent Statement: All subjects gave their informed consent for inclusion before they participated in the study.

Data Availability Statement: Supporting raw data may be obtained through special request from the corresponding author.

Acknowledgments: We thank Thomas Hocke (Cochlear Deutschland GmbH & Co. KG, Hannover, Germany) for the intellectual, administrative, and technical support in designing the experiment.

Conflicts of Interest: The institution of T.R., S.K.P. and L.W. received funding from Cochlear Research and Development Limited, Addlestone, UK, for this work and/or travel reimbursements. All other authors declare no conflicts of interest. The sponsor had no role in the execution of the study, interpretation of the results, or writing of the manuscript.

References

1. Neal, K.; McMahon, C.M.; Hughes, S.E.; Boisvert, I. Listening-Based Communication Ability in Adults With Hearing Loss: A Scoping Review of Existing Measures. *Front. Psychol.* **2022**, *13*, 786347. [CrossRef] [PubMed]
2. McRackan, T.R.; Bauschard, M.; Hatch, J.L.; Franko-Tobin, E.; Droghini, H.R.; Nguyen, S.A.; Dubno, J.R. Meta-analysis of quality-of-life improvement after cochlear implantation and associations with speech recognition abilities. *Laryngoscope* **2018**, *128*, 982–990. [CrossRef]
3. Lin, F.R.; Yaffe, K.; Xia, J.; Xue, Q.-L.; Harris, T.B.; Purchase-Helzner, E.; Satterfield, S.; Ayonayon, H.N.; Ferrucci, L.; Simonsick, E.M.; et al. Hearing loss and cognitive decline in older adults. *JAMA Intern. Med.* **2013**, *173*, 293–299. [CrossRef]
4. Livingston, G.; Huntley, J.; Sommerlad, A.; Ames, D.; Ballard, C.; Banerjee, S.; Brayne, C.; Burns, A.; Cohen-Mansfield, J.; Cooper, C.; et al. Dementia prevention, intervention, and care: 2020 report of the Lancet Commission. *Lancet* **2020**, *396*, 413–446. [CrossRef]
5. Lin, F.R.; Albert, M. Hearing loss and dementia—Who is listening? *Aging Ment. Health* **2014**, *18*, 671–673. [CrossRef]
6. Liang, Z.; Li, A.; Xu, Y.; Qian, X.; Gao, X. Hearing Loss and Dementia: A Meta-Analysis of Prospective Cohort Studies. *Front. Aging Neurosci.* **2021**, *13*, 695117. [CrossRef]
7. Weißgerber, T.; Stöver, T.; Baumann, U. Speech perception in modulated noise assessed in bimodal CI users. *HNO* **2023**, *72*, 10–16. [CrossRef]
8. Hutter, E.; Grapp, M.; Argstatter, H. Music therapy in adults with cochlear implants: Effects on music perception and subjective sound quality. *HNO* **2016**, *64*, 880–890. [CrossRef]
9. Abdel-Latif, K.H.A.; Meister, H. Speech Recognition and Listening Effort in Cochlear Implant Recipients and Normal-Hearing Listeners. *Front. Neurosci.* **2021**, *15*, 725412. [CrossRef]
10. Lundberg, E.M.H.; Strong, D.; Anderson, M.; Kaizer, A.M.; Gubbels, S. Do Patients Benefit from a Cochlear Implant When They Qualify Only in the Presence of Background Noise? *Otol. Neurotol.* **2021**, *42*, 251–259. [CrossRef]
11. Hamzavi, J.; Franz, P.; Baumgartner, W.D.; Gstöettner, W. Hearing performance in noise of cochlear implant patients versus severely-profoundly hearing-impaired patients with hearing aids. *Audiology* **2001**, *40*, 26–31. [CrossRef]
12. Mudery, J.A.; Francis, R.; McCrary, H.; Jacob, A. Older Individuals Meeting Medicare Cochlear Implant Candidacy Criteria in Noise but Not in Quiet: Are These Patients Improved by Surgery? *Otol. Neurotol.* **2017**, *38*, 187–191. [CrossRef]
13. Hey, M.; Hocke, T.; Mauger, S.; Müller-Deile, J. A clinical assessment of cochlear implant recipient performance: Implications for individualized map settings in specific environments. *Eur. Arch. Oto-Rhino-Laryngol.* **2016**, *273*, 4011–4020. [CrossRef]
14. Hey, M.; Hocke, T.; Böhnke, B.; Mauger, S.J. ForwardFocus with cochlear implant recipients in spatially separated and fluctuating competing signals—Introduction of a reference metric. *Int. J. Audiol.* **2019**, *58*, 869–878. [CrossRef] [PubMed]
15. Dawson, P.W.; Mauger, S.J.; Hersbach, A.A. Clinical evaluation of signal-to-noise ratio–based noise reduction in Nucleus®cochlear implant recipients. *Ear Hear.* **2011**, *32*, 382–390. [CrossRef] [PubMed]
16. Mauger, S.J.; Arora, K.; Dawson, P.W. Cochlear implant optimized noise reduction. *J. Neural Eng.* **2012**, *9*, 065007. [CrossRef] [PubMed]
17. Mauger, S.J.; Warren, C.D.; Knight, M.R.; Goorevich, M.; Nel, E. Clinical evaluation of the Nucleus®6 cochlear implant system: Performance improvements with SmartSound iQ. *Int. J. Audiol.* **2014**, *53*, 564–576. [CrossRef]
18. Pollack, I.; Pickett, J.M. Cocktail Party Effect. *J. Acoust. Soc. Am.* **1957**, *29*, 1262. [CrossRef]
19. Wimmer, W.; Weder, S.; Caversaccio, M.; Kompis, M. Speech Intelligibility in Noise with a Pinna Effect Imitating Cochlear Implant Processor. *Otol. Neurotol.* **2016**, *37*, 19–23. [CrossRef] [PubMed]

20. Steffens, T. The systematic selection of speech audiometric procedures. *HNO* **2017**, *65*, 219–227. [CrossRef]
21. Keidser, G.; Naylor, G.; Brungart, D.S.; Caduff, A.; Campos, J.; Carlile, S.; Carpenter, M.G.; Grimm, G.; Hohmann, V.; Holube, I.; et al. The Quest for Ecological Validity in Hearing Science: What It Is, Why It Matters, and How to Advance It. *Ear Hear.* **2020**, *41*, 5S–19S. [CrossRef]
22. Francart, T.; van Wieringen, A.; Wouters, J. Comparison of fluctuating maskers for speech recognition tests. *Int. J. Audiol.* **2011**, *50*, 2–13. [CrossRef] [PubMed]
23. Qazi, O.U.R.; van Dijk, B.; Moonen, M.; Wouters, J. Understanding the effect of noise on electrical stimulation sequences in cochlear implants and its impact on speech intelligibility. *Hear. Res.* **2013**, *299*, 79–87. [CrossRef]
24. Berg, K.A.; Noble, J.H.; Dawant, B.M.; Dwyer, R.T.; Labadie, R.F.; Gifford, R.H. Speech recognition as a function of the number of channels in perimodiolar electrode recipients. *J. Acoust. Soc. Am.* **2019**, *145*, 1556–1564. [CrossRef] [PubMed]
25. Shew, M.A.; Herzog, J.A.; Kallogjeri, D.; Chen, S.; Wick, C.; Durakovic, N.; McJunkin, J.; Buchman, C.A. The Impact of Age on Noise Sensitivity in Cochlear Implant Recipients. *Otol. Neurotol.* **2022**, *43*, 72–79. [CrossRef]
26. Füllgrabe, C. Age-dependent changes in temporal-fine-structure processing in the absence of peripheral hearing loss. *Am. J. Audiol.* **2013**, *22*, 313–315. [CrossRef]
27. Hoppe, U.; Hocke, T.; Iro, H. Age-Related Decline of Speech Perception. *Front. Aging Neurosci.* **2022**, *14*, 891202. [CrossRef]
28. Peelle, J.E. Listening Effort: How the Cognitive Consequences of Acoustic Challenge Are Reflected in Brain and Behavior. *Ear Hear.* **2018**, *39*, 204–214. [CrossRef]
29. Philips, C.; Jacquemin, L.; Lammers, M.J.W.; Mertens, G.; Gilles, A.; Vanderveken, O.M.; Van Rompaey, V. Listening effort and fatigue among cochlear implant users: A scoping review. *Front. Neurol.* **2023**, *14*, 1278508. [CrossRef]
30. Stenbäck, V.; Marsja, E.; Hällgren, M.; Lyxell, B.; Larsby, B. The Contribution of Age, Working Memory Capacity, and Inhibitory Control on Speech Recognition in Noise in Young and Older Adult Listeners. *J. Speech Lang. Hear. Res.* **2021**, *64*, 4513–4523. [CrossRef] [PubMed]
31. Perreau, A.E.; Wu, Y.-H.; Tatge, B.; Irwin, D.; Corts, D. Listening Effort Measured in Adults with Normal Hearing and Cochlear Implants. *J. Am. Acad. Audiol.* **2017**, *28*, 685–697. [CrossRef]
32. Rahne, T.; Wagner, T.M.; Kopsch, A.C.; Plontke, S.K.; Wagner, L. Influence of Age on Speech Recognition in Noise and Hearing Effort in Listeners with Age-Related Hearing Loss. *J. Clin. Med.* **2023**, *12*, 6133. [CrossRef]
33. Wagener, K.; Brand, T.; Kollmeier, B. Entwicklung und Evaluation eines Satztests für die deutsche Sprache Teil III: Evaluation des Oldenburger Satztests - Development and evaluation of a German sentence test Part III: Evaluation of the Oldenburg sentence test. *Z. Audiol.* **1999**, *38*, 86–95.
34. Kollmeier, B.; Warzybok, A.; Hochmuth, S.; Zokoll, M.A.; Uslar, V.; Brand, T.; Wagener, K.C. The multilingual matrix test: Principles, applications, and comparison across languages: A review. *Int. J. Audiol.* **2015**, *54*, 3–16. [CrossRef]
35. Krüger, M.; Schulte, M.; Holube, I. Entwicklung einer Adaptiven Skalierungsmethode zur Ermittlung der Subjektiven Höranstrengung Conference Paper, 18. Jahrestagung der Deutschen Gesellschaft für Audiologie 2015, pp. 1–6. Available online: https://www.researchgate.net/publication/277010703_Entwicklung_einer_adaptiven_Skalierungsmethode_zur_Ermittlung_der_subjektiven_Horanstrengung (accessed on 11 January 2024).
36. Rahne, T.; Fröhlich, L.; Wagner, L.; Kropp, M.H.; Müller, A. Speech perception and hearing effort using a new active middle ear implant audio processor. *Eur. Arch. Oto-Rhino-Laryngol.* **2022**, *279*, 4667–4675. [CrossRef]
37. Hey, M.; Böhnke, B.; Mewes, A.; Munder, P.; Mauger, S.J.; Hocke, T. Speech comprehension across multiple CI processor generations: Scene dependent signal processing. *Laryngoscope Investig. Otolaryngol.* **2021**, *6*, 807–815. [CrossRef]
38. Dowell, R.C. The case for earlier cochlear implantation in postlingually deaf adults. *Int. J. Audiol.* **2016**, *55*, S51–S56. [CrossRef]
39. Dazert, S.; Thomas, J.P.; Loth, A.; Zahnert, T.; Stöver, T. Cochlea-Implantation. *Dtsch. Arztebl. Int.* **2020**, *117*, 690–700. [CrossRef]
40. Badajoz-Davila, J.; Buchholz, J.M. Effect of Test Realism on Speech-in-noise Outcomes in Bilateral Cochlear Implant Users. *Ear Hear.* **2021**, *42*, 1687–1698. [CrossRef]
41. Hey, M.; Mewes, A.; Hocke, T. Speech comprehension in noise—Considerations for ecologically valid assessment of communication skills ability with cochlear implants. *HNO* **2023**, *71*, 26–34. [CrossRef]
42. Rader, T.; Fastl, H.; Baumann, U. Speech perception with combined electric-acoustic stimulation and bilateral cochlear implants in a multisource noise field. *Ear Hear.* **2013**, *34*, 324–332. [CrossRef]
43. Cooke, M. A glimpsing model of speech perception in noise. *J. Acoust. Soc. Am.* **2006**, *119*, 1562–1573. [CrossRef]
44. Rader, T.; Adel, Y.; Fastl, H.; Baumann, U. Speech Perception with Combined Electric-Acoustic Stimulation: A Simulation and Model Comparison. *Ear Hear.* **2015**, *36*, e314–e325. [CrossRef]
45. Meister, H. Speech comprehension and cognitive performance in acoustically difficult situations. *HNO* **2020**, *68*, 171–176. [CrossRef]
46. Weissgerber, T.; Stöver, T.; Baumann, U. Speech perception in noise: Impact of directional microphones in users of combined electric-acoustic stimulation. *PLoS ONE* **2019**, *14*, e0213251. [CrossRef]
47. Dreschler, W.A.; Verschuure, H.; Ludvigsen, C.; Westermann, S. ICRA noises: Artificial noise signals with speech-like spectral and temporal properties for hearing instrument assessment. *Int. J. Audiol.* **2001**, *40*, 148–157. [CrossRef]
48. Pichora-Fuller, M.K.; Kramer, S.E.; Eckert, M.A.; Edwards, B.; Hornsby, B.W.; Humes, L.E.; Lemke, U.; Lunner, T.; Matthen, M.; Mackersie, C.L.; et al. Hearing impairment and cognitive energy: The framework for understanding effortful listening (FUEL). *Ear Hear.* **2016**, *37*, 5S–27S. [CrossRef]

49. Kwak, C.; Han, W. Age-Related Difficulty of Listening Effort in Elderly. *Int. J. Environ. Res. Public Health* **2021**, *18*, 8845. [CrossRef]
50. Carlyon, R.P.; Goehring, T. Cochlear Implant Research and Development in the Twenty-first Century: A Critical Update. *J. Assoc. Res. Otolaryngol.* **2021**, *22*, 481–508. [CrossRef]

Journal of
Clinical Medicine

MDPI

Article

Outcome Prediction of Speech Perception in Quiet and in Noise for Cochlear Implant Candidates Based on Pre-Operative Measures

Tobias Weissgerber [1,*], Marcel Löschner [1], Timo Stöver [2] and Uwe Baumann [1]

[1] Audiological Acoustics, ENT Department, University Hospital, Goethe University Frankfurt, 60590 Frankfurt am Main, Germany; u.baumann@med.uni-frankfurt.de (U.B.)
[2] ENT Department, University Hospital, Goethe University Frankfurt, 60590 Frankfurt am Main, Germany
* Correspondence: weissgerber@med.uni-frankfurt.de; Tel.: +49-69-63015898

Abstract: (1) Background: The fitting of cochlear implants (CI) is an established treatment, even in cases with considerable residual hearing but insufficient speech perception. The aim of this study was to evaluate a prediction model for speech in quiet and to provide reference data and a predictive model for postoperative speech perception in noise (SPiN) after CI provision. (2) Methods: CI candidates with substantial residual hearing (either in hearing threshold or in word recognition scores) were included in a retrospective analysis ($n = 87$). Speech perception scores in quiet 12 months post-surgery were compared with the predicted scores. A generalized linear model was fitted to speech reception thresholds (SRTs) after CI fitting to identify predictive variables for SPiN. (3) Results: About two-thirds of the recipients achieved the expected outcome in quiet or were better than expected. The mean absolute error of the prediction was 13.5 percentage points. Age at implantation was the only predictive factor for SPiN showing a significant correlation ($r = 0.354$; $p = 0.007$). (4) Conclusions: Outcome prediction accuracy for speech in quiet was comparable to previous studies. For CI recipients in the included study population, the SPiN outcome could be predicted only based on the factor age.

Keywords: word recognition; speech reception threshold; generalized linear model; CI SPiN outcome

1. Introduction

In the past decades, the provision of cochlear implants (CI) has become an established therapy for patients without sufficient word recognition with hearing aids (HA) or other acoustic hearing solutions [1,2]. The expansion of indication criteria [2–4] with respect to preoperative pure-tone audiograms and aided word recognition scores (WRS) at a conversational level of 65 dB SPL, WRS_{65}(HA), and postoperative word recognition with CI, WRS_{65}(CI), improved in comparison to a patient population with poorer preoperative hearing [5,6]. Especially in subjects within the transition range between hearing aid and cochlear implant indication, e.g., with pure tone thresholds of around 60 to 80 dB and WRS_{65}(HA) scores up to 60%, an individual prediction of expected WRS_{65}(CI) is of increasing importance. In this subject population, there is a high demand for outcome prediction with CI during the consultation since they oftentimes struggle if they are potentially still "to good" for cochlear implantation and would potentially perform better with their hearing aids than with CIs.

In first attempts, some studies have shown that the preoperative maximum word recognition score, WRS_{max}, is one predicting factor for WRS_{65}(CI) [6–8]. The WRS_{max} should be exceeded by the WRS_{65}(CI) in most CI recipients. This finding is of special importance for individual counselling of CI candidates since the information-carrying capacity WRS_{max} [9] is oftentimes not achieved by using hearing aids [10–16]. Especially in the transition range between HA and CI indication, i.e., for pure-tone thresholds between 60 and 80 dB, the WRS_{65}(HA) is on average only half of the WRS_{max} in a patient cohort typically for a maximum care hospital [13]. Additionally to the WRS_{max}, recent studies found [17] and confirmed [18,19] that the age at implantation and the WRS_{65}(HA) significantly contribute to the prediction of the WRS_{65}(CI). This relation can be characterized as

$$WRS_{65}(CI)[\%] = \frac{100}{1 + e^{-(\beta_0 + \beta_1 \cdot WRS_{max} + \beta_2 \cdot Age + \beta_3 \cdot WRS_{65}(HA))}} \quad (1)$$

with $\beta_0 = 0.84 \pm 0.18$, $\beta_1 = 0.012 \pm 0.0015$, $\beta_2 = -0.0094 \pm 0.0025$ year^{-1}, and $\beta_3 = 0.0059 \pm 0.0026$; all WRS scores are expressed in %. The application of this generalized linear model (GLM) results in a prediction error (median absolute error, MAE) of 13.5 percentage points in CI recipients with a preoperative WRS_{max} larger than zero. If this measure for outcome prediction is implemented in the postoperative process, a possible mismatch between the reached and predicted WRS_{65}(CI) can have an impact on the clinical aftercare process, leading to a further decrease in the MAE down to 11.5 percentage points in this patient group [18]. Reliable prediction allows for the early identification of cases with unexpectedly poor speech perception and the start of early intervention within basic and follow-up therapy. After pathophysiological causes and technical malfunctions were excluded, CI sound processor adjustments [20], intensification of therapies, review of user behavior [21,22], and appropriate counseling [23] must be considered.

To summarize, the outcome prediction for WRS_{65}(CI) has reached a level of reliability at which it can be used in both preoperative counseling of CI candidates [17,18] and postoperative process management [18,19]. The restriction to a patient group with preoperative WRS_{max} (which is in Germany around 2/3 of most recent CI provisions [18]) led to considerable progress in outcome prediction for WRS_{65}(CI). However, to our knowledge, a similar useful outcome prediction for speech perception in noise (SPiN) based on preoperative routine data has not been established, neither in research nor in clinical routine. Additionally, CI indication criteria for WRS in quiet were formulated in all recent guidelines, e.g., [2,4,24], whereas no reliable data are yet available for speech perception in noise. However, speech perception in noise is oftentimes the main problem in everyday life. This is the main reason to ask about possible options for hearing improvement during patient counseling.

Consequently, there is a need to provide more reference data for SpiN after CI provision. Therefore, the goal of this study is to provide reference data and a predictive model for postoperative SpiN. To do so, the approach from Hoppe et al. [17,18] was used, including only CI candidates with a preoperative WRS_{max} larger than zero or substantial pure-tone residual hearing. The outcome for WRS_{65}(CI) will be compared to the predicted scores [17] to further evaluate the GLM according to Equation (1). Particularly, the SpiN, here assessed as speech reception thresholds (SRT) in noise, will be evaluated. A corresponding GLM will be derived from the data of this study. Finally, both measures will be put into relation.

2. Materials and Methods

The clinic records from 2005 to 2022 were analyzed for subjects provided with CI systems of type Nucleus Freedom or later (Cochlear, Sydney, Australia) with a preoperative WRS_{max} larger than zero or a four-frequency (test frequencies: 0.5/1/2/4 kHz) pure-tone average (4FPTA) in air conduction of better or equal 80 dB. For higher reliability of the ipsilateral post-operative free-field measures, subjects with contralateral normal hearing (i.e., single-sided deafness, SSD) were excluded. The indication criteria were fulfilled by 87 subjects (mean age: 58.3 ± 16.6 years); 30 of them used contour electrodes (5 CI24RE(CA), 11 CI512, 14 CI612); 27 subjects were implanted with straight electrodes (12 CI422, 4 CI522, 11 CI622); and 30 subjects were implanted with slim modiolar electrodes (11 CI532, 19 CI632). All study participants were provided with a CI within the current CI Guidelines [2] in Germany.

The 4FPTAs ranged between 53.8 and 102.5 dB HL (mean: 75.0 ± 8.7 dB HL), 70 of the 87 subjects had a 4FPTA better or equal to 80 dB. WRS_{max} ranged between 0% and 90% (mean: 34.0 ± 22.8%); 79 of the 87 subjects (91%) had a WRS_{max} larger than zero. The aided monosyllable score WRS_{65}(HA) (measured at 65 dB SPL, hearing aid in ipsilateral ear with contralateral masking, if necessary) ranged between 0% and 90% (mean: 21.7 ± 20.9%).

Study measures used for the prediction model pre-surgery included pure-tone audiometry (4FPTA), unaided speech audiometry in quiet (WRS_{max}), and aided speech audiometry in quiet (WRS_{65}(HA). Study measures post-surgery were speech audiometry in quiet, WRS_{65}(CI), and speech reception threshold in noise, SRT(CI).

All speech scores in quiet were assessed with the Freiburg monosyllable test [25]. Speech perception in noise was assessed with the German matrix test (Oldenburg sentence test, OlSa, [26–28]). The speech level was adaptively adjusted to measure the SRT for 50% correct word recognition, while the noise level was kept constant at 65 dB SPL. The speech and noise signals were presented from 0° azimuth. One OlSa list (20 sentences each) was used. Prior to testing, one practice list was presented to the subject to familiarize the subject with the test procedure and the speech material. The test was conducted in closed-set mode. The test subjects indicated the words on a touch-screen monitor. The test was conducted only in a unilateral setting with contralateral blocking of the ear canal and additional ear muffs (if necessary).

All included recipients were able to perform the postoperative speech in quiet test. The speech-in-noise test was completed by two-thirds of the recipients (57 of 87).

3. Results

3.1. Preoperative Pure Tone and Speech Audiometry

Figure 1a,b relate the pure-tone thresholds to WRS_{max} and WRS_{65}(HA). Figure 1c relates both word recognition scores in quiet. About 80% of the CI recipients had a preoperative 4FPTA of 80 dB or less (better). About 9% (8 of 87) of the recipients had a WRS_{max} higher than 60%. However, as illustrated in Figure 1c, these patients were not able to fully utilize this potential information-carrying capacity [9] with HA.

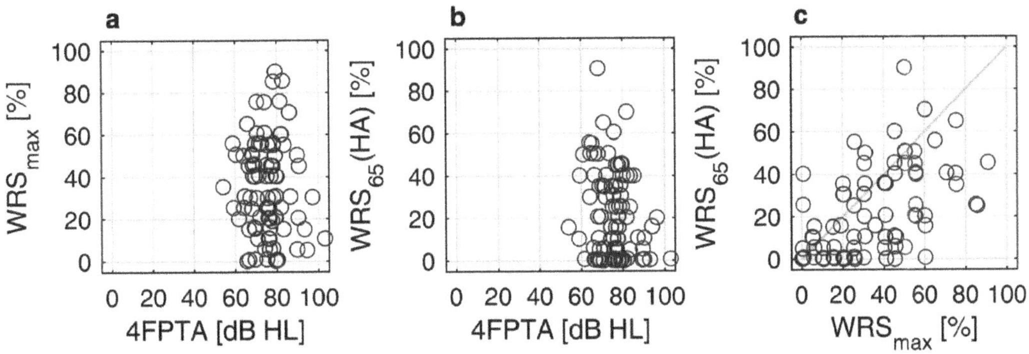

Figure 1. Scatterplots of preoperative pure-tone audiometry and speech audiometry: (**a**) Maximum word recognition score, WRS_{max}, as a function of pure tone average, 4FPTA; (**b**) Aided word recognition score, WRS_{65}(HA), as a function of 4FPTA; (**c**) Relation between WRS_{65}(HA) and WRS_{max}.

3.2. Postoperative Speech Audiometry

Figure 2a–c relate the preoperative word recognition scores WRS_{max} and WRS_{65}(HA) to the postoperative scores WRS_{65}(CI) and SRT(CI). No correlation was found between WRS_{65}(HA) and WRS_{65}(CI). A weak but significant correlation was found between WRS_{max} and WRS_{65}(CI) ($r_{spearman} = 0.226$; $p = 0.036$, Figure 2b). There was no correlation between the postoperative SRT in noise and any of the preoperative audiometric measures, neither WRS_{max}, WRS_{65}(HA) nor the 4FPTA.

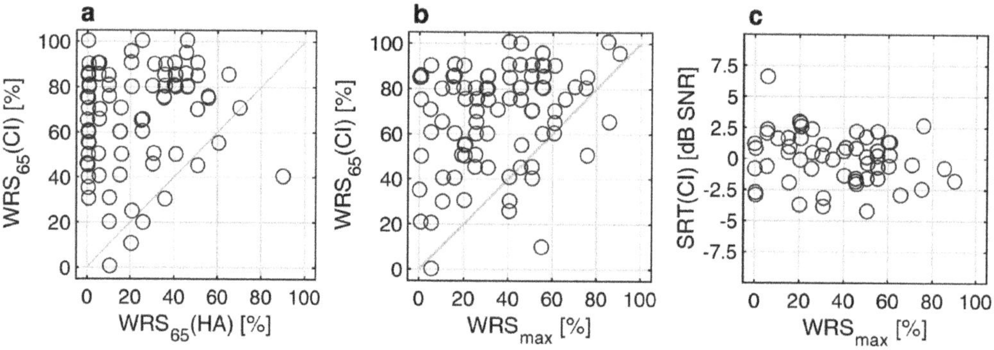

Figure 2. Postoperative pure-tone and speech audiometry after twelve months: (**a**) Word recognition score with CI, WRS_{65}(CI), as a function preoperative aided word recognition score WRS_{65}(HA); (**b**) WRS_{65}(CI) as a function of maximum word recognition score, WRS_{max}; (**c**) Relation between speech reception threshold in noise, SRT(CI), and WRS_{max}.

Within our study group with preoperative 4FPTA better or equal to 80 dB and/or WRS_{max} greater than zero, the mean improvement in word recognition scores in quiet with CI compared to HA prior to surgery was 45.9 percentage points. An improved WRS of at least 20 percentage points in 86% of all cases was observed. There was only one case with a significant decrease in word recognition after the CI provision.

3.3. *Prediction for Word Recognition in Quiet*

Figure 3a,b show the differences between measured and predicted (according to Equation (1)) WRS_{65}(CI) after twelve months. About 63% of the recipients achieved the expected outcome or were better than expected. In about 37% of the cases, there was a difference between measured and predicted scores greater than 20 percentage points (i.e., an outcome that was worse than expected). The error in WRS prediction (MAE) was 13.5 percentage points.

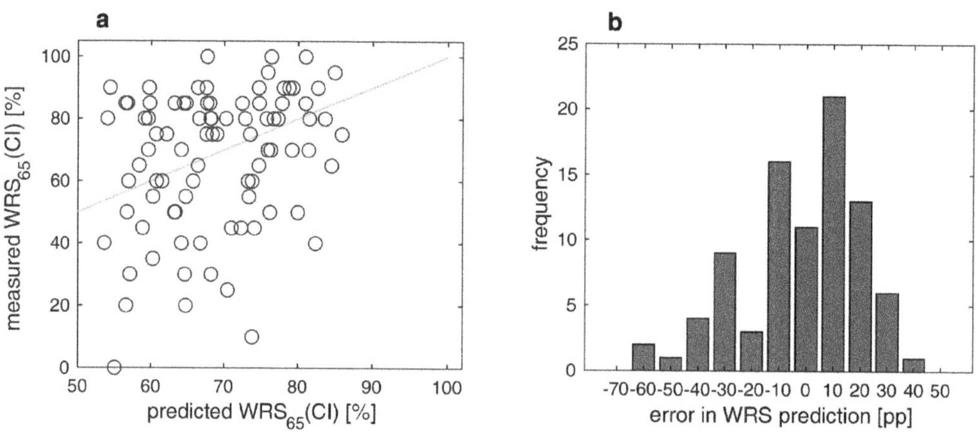

Figure 3. Measured versus predicted word recognition scores in quiet twelve months after CI surgery: (**a**) Relation between measured and predicted scores with CI, WRS_{65}(CI); (**b**) differences between measured and predicted WRS_{65}(CI). Negative/positive values correspond to poorer/better word recognition than predicted.

3.4. Prediction for Speech Recognition in Noise

A GLM was fitted to the data. In analogy to a previous study [17], WRS_{max}, WRS_{65}(HA), age, and 4FPTA were tested as predictive variables for SRT(CI). The results of the statistics of the GLM for the four tested predictive variables are summarized in Table 1.

Table 1. Results of the regression analysis (generalized linear model, GLM) with the four tested input variables (WRS_{max}, WRS_{65}(HA), age, and 4FPTA) based on twelve months data for SRT estimation.

	Estimate	Standard Error	T Statistics	p
Constant, η_0	−0.7434	2.6145	−0.2843	0.7772
WRS_{max}	−0.0030	0.0141	−0.2180	0.8282
WRS65(HA)	−0.0102	0.0147	−0.6911	0.4925
age, η_1	0.0408	0.0177	2.2976	0.0256
4FPTA	−0.0213	0.0311	−0.6857	0.4959

Included are 57 observations with 52 degrees of freedom. F-statistics vs. constant model: 3.96, p = 0.0949.

The age at implantation was the only significant contributing factor. Three of the four tested input variables do not significantly contribute to the SRT (Table 1). Consequently, the GLM has to be reduced to the one predicting variable age. This results in a GLM according to Equation (2):

$$SRT[dB] = \eta_0 + \eta_1 \cdot Age \quad (2)$$

with $\eta_0 = -2.8774 \pm 0.915$ and $\eta_1 = 0.0438 \pm 0.0161$. There was a significant correlation between age at implantation and SRT ($r_{spearman} = 0.354$; $p = 0.007$).

Figure 4a,b show the differences between measured and predicted SRTs. The largest difference was 7.6 dB. In a third of the recipients (34%), the test was not performed. The MAE was 1.3 dB. The prediction covers a range of 3.3 dB (−2.4 to 0.9 dB), while the measured SRTs differ between −4.6 and +6.4 dB.

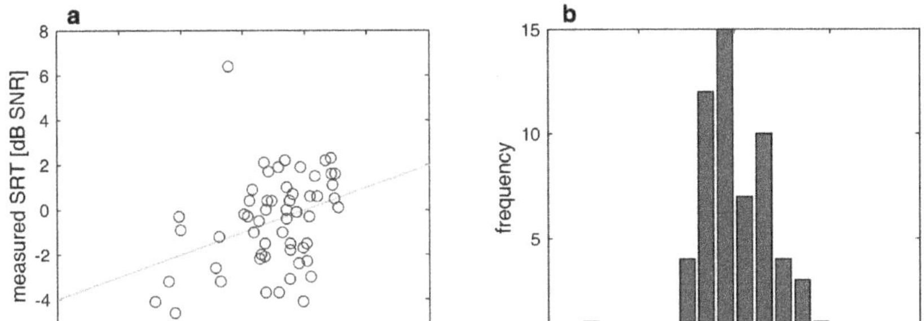

Figure 4. Measured and predicted speech recognition thresholds in noise (SRT) twelve months post-operatively: (**a**) Relation between measured and predicted SRT; (**b**) differences between measured and predicted SRT; negative/positive values correspond to poorer/better word recognition than predicted.

4. Discussion

4.1. Speech Recognition Scores in Quiet

The results of this retrospective study strongly support the indication criteria for CI provision according to the German guideline [2] in patients with considerable preoperative word recognition scores up to 60%. In our study group of CI recipients, preoperative maximum word recognition scores of up to 90% were observed. In this group, a mean improvement from WRS_{65}(HA) to WRS_{65}(CI) of 45.9 percentage points was achieved, with only one case showing a significant decrement. In 86% of all cases, speech perception in quiet with CI improved by at least 20 percentage points compared to the pre-surgery performance with a hearing aid, which is in the order of results described in other studies [29]. There was one outlier with a WRS_{65}(HA) of 90% and a WRS_{65}(CI) of 40%.

With respect to both the preoperative CI candidacy assessment [16] and the achieved postoperative results, our findings are consistent with those of other studies [7,8,17,18,29]. Overall, the measured WRS_{65}(CI) correspond to the predicted WRS_{65}(CI) with a MAE of 13.5 percentage points. Our retrospective study confirms the results of Hoppe et al. [17], who reported a MAE of 13.5 percentage points as well.

However, there were also some differences in results compared to other studies observed. The WRS_{65}(HA) did not correlate with the WRS_{65}(CI), whereas according to Hoppe and coworkers, the preoperative WRS_{65}(HA) would explain at least around 5 percentage points of the WRS_{65}(CI). The lower number of subjects (n = 87) in the present study compared to Hoppe et al. (n = 128, [17]) potentially contributed to this different finding. Furthermore, both studies slightly differ in the inclusion criteria. Hoppe et al. [17] included all recipients with 4FPTA $\leq$ 80 dB, while in our study we included all patients with 4FPTA $\leq$ 80 dB and/or $WRS_{max} > 0\%$. This resulted in around 20% of the study population showing a 4FPTA poorer than 80 dB. The rationale for this different inclusion criterion was that the 4FPTA was found to be no predictor for WRS_{65}(CI) [17]. The results of a recent study [18] also suggest that WRS_{max} is a better predictive variable than 4FPTA.

Rieck et al. [8] found no correlation between WRS_{65}(HA) and WRS_{65}(CI) but between WRS_{80}(HA) and WRS_{65}(CI). They included all adult CI patients in their analysis. There is no contradiction in the different study results since a clear and restricted definition of the study population with respect to their preoperative characteristics seems to be a key element for better outcome prediction.

4.2. Prediction Model for Speech Perception Threshold in Noise

Up to now, guidelines for CI candidacy typically only refer to speech in quiet scores [2,4,24], with some including pure-tone thresholds as a criterion [4,24]. Even though some clinics in CI candidacy evaluation already refer to SpiN performance, e.g., [4], this is not common clinical practice yet. The availability of a predictive model for SpiN could have an effect on both the preoperative candidacy evaluation and patient counseling. Furthermore, a model could impact the post-operative evaluation of hearing performance in such a way that, for example, hearing therapy is continued or intensified if hearing success is too poor compared to the prediction. As speech perception in noise is usually the main problem in everyday life for people with hearing loss, this is often the reason for them to ask about possible options for hearing improvement. Accordingly, they would also like to obtain some information during the consultation about how much SpiN could potentially be improved by the intervention. This is of special importance for subject groups with substantial residual hearing and speech perception in quiet, since they often struggle to decide on a cochlear implant due to the risk of losing their residual hearing.

To our knowledge, no model predicting SpiN (SRTs) after CI provision based on preoperative data has been published. Therefore, the aim of this work was to find a prediction model for SpiN based on pre-operative measures. A particular challenge here is that in this population, speech perception pre-surgery is usually not sufficient, such that SRTs in noise (i.e., 50% speech perception in noise) could be determined, and this potentially valuable input variable for the predictive model is not available.

The recipients in which the SRT was measured (two-thirds of all subjects) showed SRTs within a range of −4.6 to 6.4 dB. This range is comparable to the data published by Kießling et al. [30], where 75% of the CI users who were able to perform the OlSa showed SRTs of 1.3 dB SNR or lower (i.e., better). In the presented study, the SRTs of the tested subjects were better or equal to 1.3 dB SNR in 81% of the cases.

In the investigated cohort of CI recipients, certain SRTs can be expected (see Figure 4). For the SpiN prediction with CI, the regression analysis yielded a GLM with the prediction variable age, which was the only variable contributing to the SpiN prediction out of the four tested input variables: WRS_{max}, WRS_{65}(HA), 4FPTA, and age. The GLM for SRT prediction according to Equation (2) resulted in a MAE of 1.3 dB. This prediction is just slightly larger than the test-retest reliability of the Oldenburg matrix test [28].

It seems rather disappointing that the factors that already proved valuable for speech in quiet prediction do not contribute to the GLM for SpiN but only age. However, the weak correlation (r = −0.37; p = 0.004) between post-operative WRS_{65}(CI) and post-operative SRT is in accordance with this finding, showing that even after CI provision, speech performance in quiet (at least assessed with the Freiburg monosyllable test) is no reliable predictor for speech perception in noise. Cognitive deficits potentially associated with age appear to play a greater role for speech perception in noise [31,32] than for speech perception in quiet [10,13,17]. This is in line with results from Füllgrabe et al. [33] and Weissgerber et al. [34], showing a significant impact of age on speech perception even in subjects with normal hearing [33] or subjective normal hearing [34]. Weissgerber et al. reported a significant correlation between age and SRT (r = 0.539, $p < 0.001$), which was still significant after partialing out a potential high-frequency hearing loss (r = 0.44, p = 0.03).

4.3. Limitations of this Study

It must be noted that Hoppe and coworkers used post-operative data assessed 6 months after CI surgery to fit their prediction model, whereas in the present study, data obtained 12 months after surgery were compared with the prediction. The reason was that an assessment of post-operative data already at six months had potentially resulted in an even higher number of not measurable SRTs in noise. However, the observed difference between the median WRS_{65}(CI) six months (70%, [17]) and 12 months (75%, present data) after surgery was only 5 percentage points. This corresponds to a study by Holden et al. [35], which concludes that on average, about 90% of the final performance is reached after 6.3 months.

The implementation of a prediction model for SRTs in noise was restricted to only two-thirds of the patient population. For the remaining one-third of subjects, there was no SRT data after surgery available. The main reason for this is probably that the speech perception in quiet was not good enough (either measured or expected) to allow reliable convergence of the SRT to 50% speech perception. This quite high number of subjects without SRT data could also be due to the fact that the present retrospective study analyzed patient data dating back to 2005. Other studies, including more recent CI candidates with a typically better expected outcome than in the last decades, e.g., due to the shorter duration of deafness and oftentimes better residual hearing, found that the speech-in-noise test could be performed in 78% of the study population [36]. The fact that not all recipients were able to perform adaptive measurements of SRT resulted in the clinical practice of assessing speech-in-noise abilities using tests at fixed signal-to-noise ratios (typically 0 or 10 dB) [37]. This practice was discontinued by many clinics as the results improved and more patients were able to perform adaptive SRT measurements. Another aspect for predicting SpiN performance could be to use a test procedure with simpler test material as a measure, e.g., the digits-in-noise test [38]. Maybe simpler test procedures in noise could also be used as a measure and potential predictor pre-surgery in cases of sufficient residual hearing.

In the present study, the age at the date of surgery was found to be a predictor of SRT performance after CI provision. Since speech perception in noise decreases with age in even normal hearing subjects, the predictive model could be adjusted to include the age at intended testing (e.g., 6, 12, 24 months after CI provision) for performance prediction in future models. The predictive model could also be extended, including the etiology and duration of deafness as potential predictors, as these parameters were not assessed in the present work. However, etiology is oftentimes unknown, and, therefore, only a subpopulation could potentially benefit from etiology as a predictive factor. Czurda and coworkers investigated the impact of the etiology and duration of hearing loss on WRS_{65}(CI) [39]. In 60% of the 601 analyzed ears, they reported that the etiology was unknown. For the remaining subjects, they showed that etiology had a significant impact on WRS65(CI). The largest negative deviations between measured and predicted WRS65(CI) were found for the etiologies of perinatal asphyxia, Menière's disease, and trauma, with perinatal asphyxia showing the highest rate of cases (33%) missing the prognosis by more than 20 percentage points. It could be assumed that subjects with these etiologies could expect lower outcomes in WRS65(CI) than the average CI user. On the other hand, superior outcomes (i.e., better than the outcome prediction) were found in subjects with genetic hearing loss, hearing loss, and otosclerosis. In the same study, subjects were divided into two groups with a duration of hearing loss of more or less than 20 years. No significant difference in WRS_{65}(CI) was found between these two subgroups. Hoppe and co-workers included "duration of hearing impairment" and "duration of unaided hearing impairment" as model input variables for the prediction of WRS65(CI) [29]. In the subgroup of subjects with WRS_{max} greater than zero, the inclusion of both variables did not result in a lower prediction error of WRS65(CI).

5. Conclusions

The word recognition in quiet outcome in the presented study strongly supports the results found in the previous studies for outcome prediction after cochlear implantation. Different from other studies, the word recognition scores with a hearing aid prior to surgery had no impact on outcome after CI provision. For most of the CI recipients in the included study, speech perception in noise could be predicted only based on the factor age.

Author Contributions: Conceptualization, T.W. and U.B.; methodology, T.W.; validation, T.W., U.B. and T.S.; formal analysis, T.W. and M.L.; investigation, T.W. and M.L.; resources, T.W., U.B. and T.S.; data curation, T.W.; writing—original draft preparation, T.W.; writing—review and editing, T.W., U.B., T.S. and M.L.; visualization, T.W.; supervision, T.W.; project administration, T.W.; funding acquisition, T.W., U.B. and T.S.; All authors have read and agreed to the published version of the manuscript.

Funding: This work was funded by Cochlear Research and Development Ltd. (Surrey, UK), research grant number IIR-2386. The study design was done in cooperation with the funder. The funder had no role in data collection and analysis, the decision to publish, or the preparation of the manuscript. The APC was funded by Goethe University in Frankfurt.

Institutional Review Board Statement: The study was conducted in accordance with the Declaration of Helsinki and approved by the Ethics Committee of University Hospital Frankfurt (protocol code 2022-756, 24 June 2022).

Informed Consent Statement: Patient consent was waived in view of the retrospective nature of the study, and all the procedures being performed were part of routine care.

Data Availability Statement: Supporting raw data may be obtained through a special request from the corresponding author.

Acknowledgments: The authors would like to thank Thomas Hocke for fruitful discussions and comments on previous versions of the manuscript.

Conflicts of Interest: The study design was done in cooperation with the funder. The funder had no role in data collection and analysis, the decision to publish, or the preparation of the manuscript.

References

1. Buchman, C.A.; Gifford, R.H.; Haynes, D.S.; Lenarz, T.; O'Donoghue, G.; Adunka, O.; Biever, A.; Briggs, R.J.; Carlson, M.L.; Dai, P.; et al. Unilateral Cochlear Implants for Severe, Profound, or Moderate Sloping to Profound Bilateral Sensorineural Hearing Loss: A Systematic Review and Consensus Statements. *JAMA Otolaryngol. Head. Neck Surg.* **2020**, *146*, 942–953. [CrossRef]
2. AWMF. Leitlinien: Cochlea-Implantat Versorgung und Zentral-Auditorische Implantate [Guidelines: Cochlear Implant Care and Central Auditory Implants]. 2020. Available online: https://www.awmf.org/uploads/tx_szleitlinien/017-071l_S2k_Cochlea-Implantat-Versorgung-zentral-auditorische-Implantate_2020-12.pdf (accessed on 1 December 2023).
3. Gifford, R.H.; Dorman, M.F.; Shallop, J.K.; Sydlowski, S.A. Evidence for the expansion of adult cochlear implant candidacy. *Ear Hear.* **2010**, *31*, 186–194. [CrossRef] [PubMed]
4. Van der Straaten, T.F.K.; Briaire, J.J.; Vickers, D.; Boermans, P.; Frijns, J.H.M. Selection Criteria for Cochlear Implantation in the United Kingdom and Flanders: Toward a Less Restrictive Standard. *Ear Hear.* **2020**, *42*, 68–75. [CrossRef] [PubMed]
5. Helbig, S.; Adel, Y.; Rader, T.; Stover, T.; Baumann, U. Long-term Hearing Preservation Outcomes After Cochlear Implantation for Electric-Acoustic Stimulation. *Otol. Neurotol.* **2016**, *37*, e353–e359. [CrossRef] [PubMed]

6. Hoppe, U.; Hocke, T.; Hast, A.; Iro, H. Maximum preimplantation monosyllabic score as predictor of cochlear implant outcome. *HNO* **2019**, *67*, 62–68. [CrossRef] [PubMed]
7. Thangavelu, K.; Nitzge, M.; Weiß, R.M.; Mueller-Mazzotta, J.; Stuck, B.A.; Reimann, K. Role of cochlear reserve in adults with cochlear implants following post-lingual hearing loss. *Eur. Arch. Otorhinolaryngol.* **2022**, *280*, 1063–1071. [CrossRef] [PubMed]
8. Rieck, J.H.; Beyer, A.; Mewes, A.; Caliebe, A.; Hey, M. Extended Preoperative Audiometry for Outcome Prediction and Risk Analysis in Patients Receiving Cochlear Implants. *J. Clin. Med.* **2023**, *12*, 3262. [CrossRef] [PubMed]
9. Halpin, C.; Rauch, S. Clinical implications of a damaged cochlea: Pure tone thresholds vs. information-carrying capacity. *Otolaryngol.-Head Neck Surg.* **2009**, *140*, 473–476. [CrossRef]
10. Hoppe, U.; Hast, A.; Hocke, T. Sprachverstehen mit Hörgeraten in Abhängigkeit vom Tongehör [Speech recognition with hearing aids depending on pure-tone hearing]. *HNO* **2014**, *62*, 443–448. [CrossRef]
11. McRackan, T.R.; Ahlstrom, J.B.; Clinkscales, W.B.; Meyer, T.A.; Dubno, J.R. Clinical Implications of Word Recognition Differences in Earphone and Aided Conditions. *Otol. Neurotol.* **2016**, *37*, 1475–1481. [CrossRef]
12. McRackan, T.R.; Fabie, J.E.; Burton, J.A.; Munawar, S.; Holcomb, M.A.; Dubno, J.R. Earphone and Aided Word Recognition Differences in Cochlear Implant Candidates. *Otol. Neurotol.* **2018**, *39*, e543–e549. [CrossRef] [PubMed]
13. Kronlachner, M.; Baumann, U.; Stover, T.; Weissgerber, T. Investigation of the quality of hearing aid provision in seniors considering cognitive functions. *Laryngorhinootologie* **2018**, *97*, 852–859. [CrossRef] [PubMed]
14. Franks, Z.G.; Jacob, A. The speech perception gap in cochlear implant patients. *Cochlear Implant. Int.* **2019**, *20*, 176–181. [CrossRef] [PubMed]
15. Dörfler, C.; Hocke, T.; Hast, A.; Hoppe, U. Speech recognition with hearing aids for 10 standard audiograms: English version. *HNO* **2020**, *68*, 93–99. [CrossRef] [PubMed]
16. Beyer, A.; Rieck, J.H.; Mewes, A.; Dambon, J.A.; Hey, M. Extended preoperative speech audiometric diagnostics for cochlear implant treatment. *HNO* **2023**, *71*, 779–786. [CrossRef] [PubMed]
17. Hoppe, U.; Hocke, T.; Hast, A.; Iro, H. Cochlear Implantation in Candidates With Moderate-to-Severe Hearing Loss and Poor Speech Perception. *Laryngoscope* **2021**, *131*, e940–e945. [CrossRef] [PubMed]
18. Hoppe, U.; Hast, A.; Hocke, T. Validation of a predictive model for speech discrimination after cochlear implant provision. *HNO* **2023**, *71*, 53–59. [CrossRef]
19. Dziemba, O.C.; Merz, S.; Hocke, T. Evaluative audiometry after cochlear implant provision. *HNO* **2023**, *72*, 56–62. [CrossRef]
20. Rader, T.; Doms, P.; Adel, Y.; Weissgerber, T.; Strieth, S.; Baumann, U. A method for determining precise electrical hearing thresholds in cochlear implant users. *Int. J. Audiol.* **2018**, *57*, 502–509. [CrossRef]
21. Busch, T.; Vanpoucke, F.; Van Wieringen, A. Auditory Environment Across the Life Span of Cochlear Implant Users: Insights From Data Logging. *J. Speech Lang. Hear. Res.* **2017**, *60*, 1362–1377. [CrossRef]
22. Oberhoffner, T.; Hoppe, U.; Hey, M.; Hecker, D.; Bagus, H.; Voigt, P.; Schicktanz, S.; Braun, A.; Hocke, T. Multicentric analysis of the use behavior of cochlear implant users. *Laryngorhinootologie* **2018**, *97*, 313–320. [CrossRef]
23. Glaubitz, C.; Liebscher, T.; Hoppe, U. Children with cochlear implant and additional disabilities benefit from consistent device use. *Int. J. Pediatr. Otorhinolaryngol.* **2022**, *162*, 111301. [CrossRef] [PubMed]
24. National Institute for Health and Care Excellence. Cochlear Implants for Children and Adults with Severe to Profound Deafness. 2019. Available online: https://www.nice.org.uk/guidance/ta566 (accessed on 1 December 2023).
25. Hahlbrock, K.H. *Sprachaudiometrie—Grundlagen und praktische Anwendung Einer Sprachaudiometrie für das Deutsche Sprachgebiet [Speech Audiometry—Basics and Practical Application of Speech Audiometry for the German Language Area]*; Georg Thieme Verlag: Stuttgart, Germany, 1957.
26. Wagener, K.C.; Kühnel, V.; Kollmeier, B. Entwicklung und Evaluation eines Satztests für die deutsche Sprache I: Design des Oldenburger Satztests [Development and evaluation of a sentence test for the German language I: Design of the Oldenburg sentence test]. *Z. Für Audiol.* **1999**, *1*, 4–15.
27. Wagener, K.C.; Kühnel, V.; Kollmeier, B. Entwicklung und Evaluation eines Satztests für die deutsche Sprache II: Optimierung des Oldenburger Satztests [Development and evaluation of a sentence test for the German language II: Optimization of the Oldenburg sentence test]. *Z. Für Audiol.* **1999**, *2*, 44–56.
28. Wagener, K.C.; Kühnel, V.; Kollmeier, B. Entwicklung und Evaluation eines Satztests für die deutsche Sprache III: Evaluation des Oldenburger Satztests [Development and evaluation of a sentence test for the German language III: Evaluation of the Oldenburg sentence test]. *Z. Für Audiol.* **1999**, *3*, 86–95.
29. Hoppe, U.; Hast, A.; Hornung, J.; Hocke, T. Evolving a Model for Cochlear Implant Outcome. *J. Clin. Med.* **2023**, *12*, 6215. [CrossRef] [PubMed]
30. Kießling, J.; Kollmeier, B.; Baumann, U. *Versorgung mit Hörgeräten und Hörimplantaten [Provision of Hearing Aids and Hearing Implants]*, 3rd ed.; Georg Thieme Verlag: Stuttgart, Germany, 2018.
31. Dryden, A.; Allen, H.A.; Henshaw, H.; Heinrich, A. The Association Between Cognitive Performance and Speech-in-Noise Perception for Adult Listeners: A Systematic Literature Review and Meta-Analysis. *Trends Hear.* **2017**, *21*, 2331216517744675. [CrossRef] [PubMed]
32. Gundogdu, O.; Serbetcioglu, M.B.; Kara, E.; Eser, B.N. Effects of Cognitive Functions on Speech Recognition in Noise in Cochlear Implant Recipients. *ORL J. Otorhinolaryngol. Relat. Spec.* **2023**, *85*, 208–214. [CrossRef]

33. Füllgrabe, C.; Moore, B.C.; Stone, M.A. Age-group differences in speech identification despite matched audiometrically normal hearing: Contributions from auditory temporal processing and cognition. *Front. Aging Neurosci.* **2014**, *6*, 347. [CrossRef]
34. Weissgerber, T.; Müller, C.; Stöver, T.; Baumann, U. Age Differences in Speech Perception in Noise and Sound Localization in Individuals With Subjective Normal Hearing. *Front. Psychol.* **2022**, *13*, 845285. [CrossRef]
35. Holden, L.K.; Finley, C.C.; Firszt, J.B.; Holden, T.A.; Brenner, C.; Potts, L.G.; Gotter, B.D.; Vanderhoof, S.S.; Mispagel, K. Heydebrand, G.; et al. Factors affecting open-set word recognition in adults with cochlear implants. *Ear Hear.* **2013**, *34*, 342–360 [CrossRef]
36. Hoppe, U.; Hocke, T.; Digeser, F. Bimodal benefit for cochlear implant listeners with different grades of hearing loss in the opposite ear. *Acta Otolaryngol.* **2018**, *138*, 713–721. [CrossRef]
37. Hochmair-Desoyer, I.; Schulz, E.; Moser, L.; Schmidt, M. The HSM sentence test as a tool for evaluating the speech understanding in noise of cochlear implant users. *Am. J. Otol.* **1997**, *18*, S83.
38. Smits, C.; Theo Goverts, S.; Festen, J.M. The digits-in-noise test: Assessing auditory speech recognition abilities in noise. *J. Acoust. Soc. Am.* **2013**, *133*, 1693–1706. [CrossRef]
39. Czurda, R.; Wesarg, T.; Aschendorff, A.; Beck, R.L.; Hocke, T.; Ketterer, M.C.; Arndt, S. Investigation of Maximum Monosyllabic Word Recognition as a Predictor of Speech Understanding with Cochlear Implant. *J. Clin. Med.* **2024**, *13*, 646. [CrossRef]

Journal of
Clinical Medicine

MDPI

Article

Influence of Age on Speech Recognition in Noise and Hearing Effort in Listeners with Age-Related Hearing Loss

Torsten Rahne *,†, Telse M. Wagner †, Anna C. Kopsch , Stefan K. Plontke and Luise Wagner

Department of Otorhinolaryngology, University Medicine Halle, Ernst-Grube-Straße 40, 06120 Halle (Saale), Germany; telse.wagner@gmail.com (T.M.W.)
* Correspondence: torsten.rahne@uk-halle.de
† These authors contributed equally to this work.

Abstract: The aim of this study was to measure how age affects the speech recognition threshold (SRT_{50}) of the Oldenburg Sentence Test (OLSA) and the listening effort at the corresponding signal-to-noise ratio (SNR_{cut}). The study also investigated the effect of the spatial configuration of sound sources and noise signals on SRT_{50} and SNR_{cut}. To achieve this goal, the study used olnoise and icra5 noise presented from one or more spatial locations from the front and back. Ninety-nine participants with age-related hearing loss in the 18–80 years age range, specifically in the 18–30, 31–40, 41–50, 51–60, 61–70, and 71–80 age groups, participated in this study. Speech recognition and listening effort in noise were measured and compared between the different age groups, different spatial sound configurations and noise signals. Speech recognition in noise decreased with age and became significant from the age group of 50–51. The decrease in SRT_{50} with age was greater for icra5 noise than for olnoise. For all age groups, SRT_{50} and SNR_{cut} were better for icra5 noise than for olnoise. The measured age-related reference data for SRT_{50} and SNR_{cut} can be used in further studies in listeners with age-related hearing loss and hearing aid or implant users.

Keywords: hearing in noise; age-related hearing loss; reference values; hearing effort; speech recognition

1. Introduction

Human hearing typically deteriorates with age. Regarding the correlation of the age-related decline in outer hair cells and later in inner hair cells, the pure-tone hearing thresholds are negatively affected. In addition to pure-tone hearing loss, speech recognition thresholds in noise increase with age and may be correlated with reduced outer hair cell function [1]. Even individuals with normal pure-tone hearing thresholds (i.e., normal hearing listeners) may experience reduced speech recognition in noise with age [2], which may be caused by cognitive decline. Both peripheral dysfunction and cognitive factors contribute to age-related hearing loss and communication deficits, and are difficult to disentangle.

To assess speech recognition in noisy environments in relation to age, the HÖRSTAT study examined 1903 adults using the Göttingen Sentence Test (GÖSA) and pure-tone audiometry. The study found a gradual decline in pure-tone and speech recognition thresholds (SRTs) as age increases [2]. As part of the UK Biobank, around 500,000 individuals aged 40–69 years were evaluated for speech-in-noise hearing and cognition. The data show that speech-in-noise hearing decreases exponentially with age after the age of approximately 50. This contrasts with earlier audiogram data, which indicate a more linear decline in men under 40 years and consistently less hearing loss in women [3].

The decline in the ability to understand speech in older listeners cannot be solely attributed to the effects of aging on the auditory periphery and cognition [4,5]. Furthermore, cognitive abilities play a significant role in understanding speech in noisy settings [6,7]. It is important to take into account the contributions of central auditory processing at the brainstem and cortical levels. According to the hypothesis, age-related alterations in the balance between inhibitory and excitatory neural mechanisms modify the production of gamma oscillations, thereby influencing perceptual binding [8]. Consequently, speech comprehension in noisy environments is also affected. Among older adults, central auditory processing at the level of sensation, as indicated by sensory gating, has a minimal effect on speech recognition in noise. However, it significantly impacts perceptual organization [8].

Although hearing loss and age have been identified as the main contributors to decreased speech recognition in noisy environments [9], hearing in noise deficits could also start from an early age. There are also non-speech psychoacoustic aspects to consider, like dichotic signal detection, multi-burst masking, stream segregation, and modulation detection influencing speech recognition in noise, even when hearing aids are employed [10]. In a study carried out on young and elderly people with normal hearing conditions, Füllgrabe and Moore [11] proved that there is a strong correlation between the understanding of speech in noisy environments and sensitivity to temporal fine structures.

Speech perception in noise can be assessed using matrix sentence tests [12]. The Oldenburg Sentence Test (OLSA, HoerTech, Oldenburg, Germany) is a commonly used matrix test available for several languages, and it is accessible for clinical use [12–14]. It enables the evaluation of speech intelligibility in noisy scenarios for people with different levels of hearing loss. It includes a variety of noise signals that can be utilised to generate complex listening conditions with multiple sources of speech and noise. Various noise signals are utilised in clinical practice and research to measure speech reception thresholds (SRTs). Noise that has the same spectrum as speech (e.g., the olnoise employed in the OLSA) can provide effective masking. The SRT measured in fluctuating noise can be higher than that measured in stationary noise [15]. Weißgerber et al. [16] conducted a study on amplitude-modulated Fastl noise and assessed the speech recognition of a group of bimodal cochlear implant users, comparing their results to age-matched hearing aid users, individuals without subjective hearing loss, and a young normal hearing control group. The researchers observed that speech recognition in modulated noise was more considerably impacted than in continuous noise with an increase in hearing loss. In this study, olnoise generated by a male speaker and icra5 noise, which simulates speech with pauses, were used. The icra5 noise was originally developed using live English speech from the EUROM database by the International Collegium of Rehabilitative Audiology (ICRA) [17].

In clinical practice, speech recognition in noisy situations is measured using various parameters. The number and spatial positioning of speech and noise sources, as well as the type of speech material and adaptive procedures used, can all vary between measurements of speech recognition in noise [18–20]. This makes it difficult to compare results, due to the absence of reference data for individuals with normal age-related hearing across different age groups. For the first time, Decambron et al.'s study [21] has presented objective signal-to-noise ratio (SNR) values for varied age cohorts. The study assessed the 50% speech recognition threshold (SRT_{50}) in noise via the 'Vocale Rapide dans le Bruit' test among 200 patients. The exam incorporated five noise sources with frontal speech presentation. The median values for SRT ranged from −0.37 dB (SNR) for those aged between 20–30 years to 6.84 dB (SNR) for individuals above 70 years of age. Mukari et al. [22] conducted a study on speech recognition in noisy environments using the Hearing in Noise Test (HINT). The researchers compared the Speech Reception Threshold (SRT) values obtained from three different noise sources: frontal, right and left. The study found evidence of an age-related decline in speech recognition ability, with older adults demonstrating poorer performance. Additionally, the research indicates that hearing thresholds have a significant impact on speech recognition ability in quiet conditions for older adults. However, it indicates that additional factors, including central auditory processing and cognitive abilities, could be more significant determinants in speech recognition performance in noisy environments.

In addition to assessing speech perception in noisy conditions, it is also important to evaluate listening effort. Active listening requires cognitive resources such as focus and attention. Decreased speech levels in quiet environments or the Signal-to-Noise Ratio (SNR) in noisy situations increase the demand on cognitive resources [23]. It is anticipated that age-related drops in pure-tone thresholds or hearing deficits beyond will lead to heightened listening effort, which may subsequently impact numerous daily communication scenarios with greater demands [23]. Listening effort increases with age regardless of hearing sensitivity [24]. According to the study by Kwak and Han [25], older adults experience a greater amount of listening effort compared to younger people as a result of background noise, directionality and ageing. A direct correlation was found between participants' listening effort and their working memory and processing speed performance whilst understanding speech in background noise. Thus, it can be inferred that older adults require more cognitive resources to comprehend speech in such conditions [26].

Listening effort can be measured objectively by pupillometry. However, it was observed that pupil dilatation was less affected by SNR variation than subjective measures of listening effort [27]. The Adaptive Categorical Listening Effort Scaling Test (ACALES) is a subjective clinical procedure that has recently emerged offering an excellent means of measuring listening effort in noisy environments [24]. The sentential stimuli are presented alongside varying levels of background noise, quantified by signal-to-noise ratios (SNRs). The evaluation of listening effort is based on subjective responses and utilises either a 7-point or 14-point categorical scale that spans from a 'no effort' response to one indicating 'extreme effort'. The SNRs of ACALES are adjusted presentation-by-presentation, based on prior subjective ratings. This guarantees comprehensive coverage across all possible categories and ultimately determines the moderate-level listening effort SNR_{cut} [26,28]. ACALES has been effectively employed to measure listening effort in individuals with hearing implants within a challenging acoustic environment [18,20].

This study aimed to evaluate the influence of age on the SRT_{50} of the Oldenburg sentence test (OLSA). For the first time, reference values for different age groups will be provided, including different spatial speech and noise configurations as well as noise signals. Noise will be presented in front (S_0N_0; reference and training condition) or behind (S_0N_{180}), as well as in a semicircle in front ($S_0N_{0,45,-45}$) or behind ($S_0N_{135,180,-135}$) of the participant. The study also examined for the first time how age affects listening effort when hearing in noisy environments.

2. Materials and Methods

This study consisted of exploratory cohorts and was prospective and non-interventional. It focused on adult volunteers with age- and sex-related pure-tone thresholds. The subjects were recruited in Halle (Saale), Germany, through personal contacts of the authors. The inclusion criteria required age-related hearing in both ears, fluency in German (native speakers), and to be between 18 and 80 years of age. Age-related hearing was confirmed when the bilateral pure-tone thresholds for air-conduction, averaged over 0.5, 1, 2, and 4 kHz (4PTA), were not worse than the age- and sex-related 95th percentile of the ISO 7026 [29] and there was symmetry between both ears. The Freiburg Monosyllables Test was used to measure the Word Recognition Score (WRS) of both ears, at a sound pressure level of 65 dB via headphones. Audiological evaluations were performed using an AT100 audiometer (Auritec, Hamburg, Germany).

Participants were excluded if they were unable to visit the study site, lacked fluency in the German language, demonstrated a lack of comprehension of the study procedures (also to ensure mental health), were pregnant, or did not meet the inclusion criteria. Informed written consent was obtained from all participants for their participation in the study. The study was conducted at the Audiology Lab of University Medicine Halle, Germany, after receiving ethical approval from the Medical Faculty of the Martin Luther University Halle-Wittenberg (approval number 2021-044) and was conducted in compliance with the Declaration of Helsinki.

The participants were selected from six age categories (18–30, 31–40, 41–50, 51–60, 61–70, 71–80 years). The sample size was calculated assuming an alpha of 0.05 and a power of 80%. The slope of the speech discrimination function at the reflection point, i.e., the SRT_{50}, was about 17% per dB [13]. For sample size estimation in this study, a difference of at least 2 dB (SD = 2 dB) was considered necessary to account for a relevant SRT_{50} difference. Therefore, each age required at least 16 participants in the sample size.

For testing speech recognition in noisy environments, the German Matrix Sentence Test OLSA (Hörtech, Oldenburg, Germany) was used, which was played through four loudspeakers. Signal generation and presentation were conducted using the Oldenburger Measurement Application 2.2 R&D software from Hörtech in Oldenburg, Germany, along with a Gigaport eX audio interface from ESI Audiotechnik in Leonberg, Germany, and a PLMRA400 amplifier from Pyle in Brooklyn, NY, USA. Continuous noise signals were presented at a sound pressure level of 65 dB. The stimuli utilised were either the generic noise of the Oldenburg Logatome Speech Corpus with a male voice (olnoise) or the icra5 noise. Lists of 20 sentences were presented in front (S_0N_0; reference and training condition) or behind (S_0N_{180}), as well as in a semicircle in front ($S_0N_{0,45,-45}$) or behind ($S_0N_{135,180,-135}$), of the participant, all at a distance of 1 metre from the head centre (refer to Figure 1). In clinical practice, many different spatial configurations of speech and noise sources are used. Since many hearing aid or cochlear implant algorithms aim for a better understanding of speech coming from the front and to mitigate noise coming from frontal and other directions, we focus on speech coming from the front in this study. This is also relevant for the elderly who are to be included in this study. For each sentence, the sound pressure level was adjusted based on the participant's response to the preceding sentence. This technique was performed to measure the open-set speech recognition threshold (SRT) for 50% correct recognition (SRT_{50}), which was the primary endpoint for the S_0N_0 condition using olnoise, as well as a secondary endpoint for all other spatial conditions and the icra5 noise.

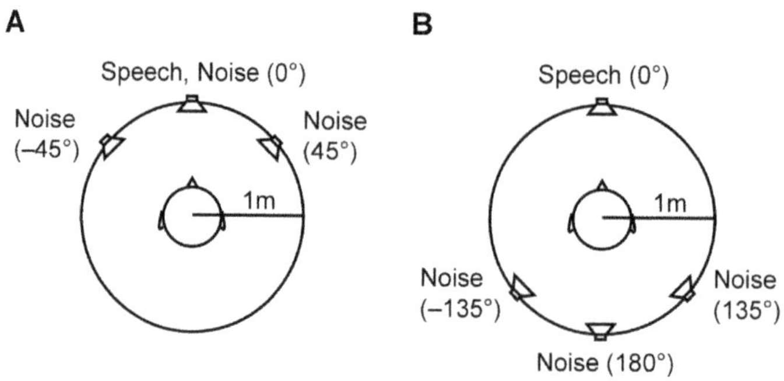

Figure 1. Experimental setup for speech and noise presentation. Speech signals were presented frontally, while noise signals were presented in a frontal (**A**) or backward (**B**) configuration.

Listening effort was assessed utilizing ACALES v2.2 software (Hörtech, Oldenburg, Germany). The participants received a sequence of two consecutive sentences from the OLSA, with diverse signal-to-noise ratios (SNRs), presented frontally, in a background noise continuously played at 65 dB SPL (either olnoise or icra5) either from the frontal (S_0N_0) or rear (S_0N_{180}) loudspeaker after two training runs. Following the presentation of two OLSA sentences in noise, participants were instructed to rate their listening effort on a scale of eight response categories, ranging from 'no effort' to 'only noise'. The signal-to-noise ratio (SNR) was changed adaptively for every round of two sentences, based on the previous assessment of the subjectively perceived listening effort, and was presented at a different SNR ranging between −40 dB and +20 dB. A listening effort function was computed by the software. The SNR_{cut}, which represents the signal-to-noise ratio (SNR) at which a moderate effort was measured (called SNR_{cut}), was assessed as a secondary endpoint for all experimental conditions by identifying the cutting point at 4 ESCU.

All the participants were seated and their heads were immobilised with a Papillon head fixation system (Focal Meditech, Tilburg, The Netherlands). After completing two

OLSA and two ACALES training sessions, all participants accomplished 15 testing runs in which the noise signals and spatial conditions were applied in a pseudorandom sequence.

The primary and secondary endpoints were analysed descriptively in this exploratory study and normality was assessed using the Shapiro–Wilk test. An ANOVA for repeated measures was used to compare the distributions of SRT_{50} and SNR_{cut} across both the 'noise signal' and 'spatial configuration' experimental conditions, as well as the 'age group' factor among subjects. Mauchly's test was used to verify the assumption of sphericity. The Bonferroni correction was employed to adjust degrees of freedom for all post hoc comparisons. Statistical analyses were conducted using version 28 of the SPSS software (IBM, Ehningen, Germany). Linear regression analysis was performed to measure the influence of the variables 'age' and 'binaurally averaged PTA' on the SRT_{50} and SNR_{cut}.

3. Results

All participants successfully completed the experiment. The demographic data of participants from all age groups are presented in Table 1. Figure 2 provides a comparison of SRT_{50} and SNR_{cut} across all spatial configurations of signal and noise sources for all participants. All spatial conditions demonstrated a better SRT_{50} and reduced listening effort for icra5 noise compared to olnoise.

Table 1. Demographic data.

Characteristics	Age Group, Years					
	18–30	**31–40**	**41–50**	**51–60**	**61–70**	**71–80**
Number	18	16	15	18	16	16
Age, mean (SD), years	24.6 (3.9)	34.5 (2.7)	46.8 (2.7)	53.0 (1.5)	66.2 (2.9)	75.8 (2.9)
Men/women, N	14/4	13/3	8/7	12/6	12/6	13/3
Hearing, mean (SD), dB PTA						
Right ear	8.0 (4.7)	8.3 (3.6)	13.3 (5.2)	17.1 (7.4)	22.3 (9.5)	25.9 (8.8)
Median [25th, 75th percentiles]	7.5 [5.0,10.0]	6.9 [6.3,11.3]	13.8 [10.0,17.5]	15.6 [11.3,20.0]	19.4 [15.0,29.7]	25.3 [19.4,34.1]
Left ear	6.8 (5.1)	8.4 (4.5)	14.1 (5.1)	17.1 (6.4)	22.6 (8.2)	27.3 (11.2)
Median [25th, 75th percentiles]	6.3 [3.8,7.5]	7.5 [5.0,12.2]	11.3 [10.0,18.8]	15.6 [12.2,22.8]	22.5 [13.1,28.8]	30.0 [17.8,36.9]
Average over both ears	7.5 (5.3)	8.5 (3.8)	14.4 (4.5)	17.5 (6.8)	23.1 (8.4)	26.6 (9.7)
Median [25th, 75th percentiles]	6.8 [4.4,9.4]	8.8 [5.6,11.3]	14.1 [10.5,18.3]	17.2 [12.5,20.8]	21.3 [15.0,30.0]	27.8 [18.6,35.6]
Word recognition, mean (SD), % correct @ 65dB SPL						
Right ear	99.0 (2.1)	99.0 (2.1)	97.9 (3.2)	96.3 (4.3)	88.3 (14.4)	87.8 (8.2)
Median [25th, 75th percentiles]	100 [100,100]	100 [100,100]	100 [95,100]	95 [95,100]	95 [80,100]	90 [81.3,93,8]
Left ear	99.0 (2.8)	98.3 (3.1)	98.2 (2.5)	96.6 (5.7)	90.0 (11.6)	84.0 (13.8)
Median [25th, 75th percentiles]	100 [100,100]	100 [95,100]	100 [95,100]	100 [95,100]	95 [80,100]	87.5 [72.5,95]

Abbreviations: SD: standard deviation; dB $PTA_{0.5\text{-}4}$: Decibel pure tone average over 0.5, 1, 2, and 4 kHz; SPL: Sound pressure level.

The box plots in Figure 3 depict the SRT_{50} distributions across all age groups. Table 2 provides the specific means and standard deviations for all conditions. The ANOVA conducted on the SRT_{50} distribution demonstrated significant main effects of noise signal ($F(1,89) = 1730.8$, $p < 0.001$), spatial configuration ($F(2.41,223.5) = 488.5$, $p < 0.001$) and the between-subjects factor of age group ($F(5,89) = 270.3$, $p < 0.001$). Interactions between the noise signal and age group ($F(5) = 18.3$, $p < 0.001$), spatial configuration and age group ($F(12.6) = 2.1$, $p < 0.01$), noise signal and spatial configuration ($F(2.43,216.6) = 738.9$, $p < 0.001$) and noise signal and spatial configuration $\times$ age group ($F(12.2) = 3.35$, $p < 0.001$)

were also significant. The post hoc comparison showed a better (lower) SRT_{50} for icra5 noise than for olnoise overall and in all age groups. The mean SRT_{50} was lowest (best) for the S_0N_{180} presentation, significantly different between all spatial configurations with an increase to $S_0N_{180,135,-135}$, S_0N_0 and $S_0N_{0,45,-45}$. The post hoc comparison showed a significant increase between the age groups 18–50 and 61–80 years when olnoise was used. However, when icra5 noise was used, the difference was significant between the age groups 18–30 years, 51–80 years and between the age groups 31–50 years and 61–80 years.

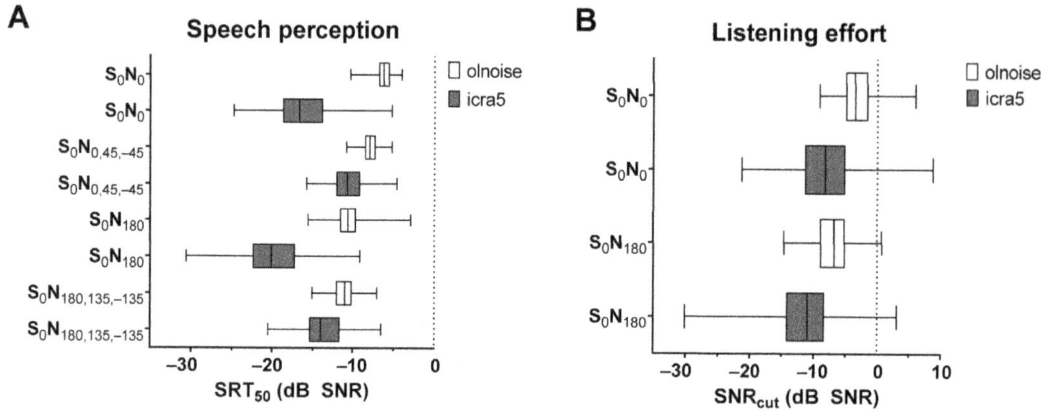

Figure 2. Speech recognition (**A**) and listening effort (**B**) in noise for all spatial conditions with olnoise (white) or icra5 noise (grey), presented as box plots (median, min, max), for all included participants.

Table 2. Outcome measures of speech perception and listening effort in noise.

Outcome	Age Group, Years					
	18–30	31–40	41–50	51–60	61–70	71–80
Speech perception in noise						
SRT_{50} in dB SNR, mean (SD)						
Olnoise, S_0N_0	−6.64 (0.75)	−6.53 (0.65)	−6.54 (0.58)	−6.18 (0.78)	−5.95 (1.38)	−4.91 (0.60)
Olnoise, S_0N_{180}	−11.43 (1.58)	−11.11 (1.63)	−11.19 (1.62)	−10.46 (2.32)	−9.75 (1.48)	−9.54 (1.84)
Olnoise, $S_0N_{0,45,-45}$	−8.51 (0.74)	−8.19 (0.85)	−8.14 (0.60)	−7.74 (0.71)	−7.10 (0.87)	−6.91 (0.91)
Olnoise, $S_0N_{180,135,-135}$	−12.35 (1.58)	−11.57 (1.26)	−11.06 (1.47)	−11.04 (1.11)	−10.40 (1.38)	−10.23 (1.69)
Icra5, S_0N_0	−18.53 (2.67)	−18.66 (2.27)	−17.39 (1.73)	−16.39 (2.28)	−14.11 (3.47)	−11.60 (2.37)
Icra5, S_0N_{180}	−22.52 (2.34)	−21.41 (2.81)	−20.44 (3.05)	−19.98 (2.58)	−16.87 (3.10)	−15.78 (3.53)
Icra5, $S_0N_{0,45,-45}$	−12.41 (1.27)	−11.89 (1.68)	−11.01 (1.52)	−1.13 (1.37)	−9.25 (1.78)	−7.95 (1.77)
Icra5, $S_0N_{180,135,-135}$	−16.20 (1.74)	−14.67 (1.75)	−14.26 (1.95)	−13.34 (1.57)	−12.33 (2.05)	−11.20 (2.25)
Listening effort in noise						
SNR_{cut} in dB SNR, mean (SD)						
Olnoise, S_0N_0	−3.2 (2.4)	−2.5 (2.6)	−2.4 (1.8)	−2.5 (3.0)	−3.6 (2.1)	−4.6 (2.5)
Olnoise, S_0N_{180}	−7.9 (2.6)	−5.8 (3.6)	−6.8 (3.6)	−6.8 (3.5)	−8.2 (3.1)	−7.6 (2.4)
Icra5, S_0N_0	−10.3 (4.6)	−7.6 (4.1)	−7.9 (3.9)	−6.8 (5.1)	−9.1 (5.4)	−8.7 (4.4)
Icra5, S_0N_{180}	−13.5 (4.4)	−10.4 (4.9)	−10.6 (3.7)	−10.7 (5.8)	−12.8 (4.5)	−12.0 (6.0)

Abbreviations: SD: standard deviation; SRT_{50}: 50% speech reception threshold, SNR: signal-to-noise ration; SNR_{cut}: signal to noise ratio at moderate listening effort.

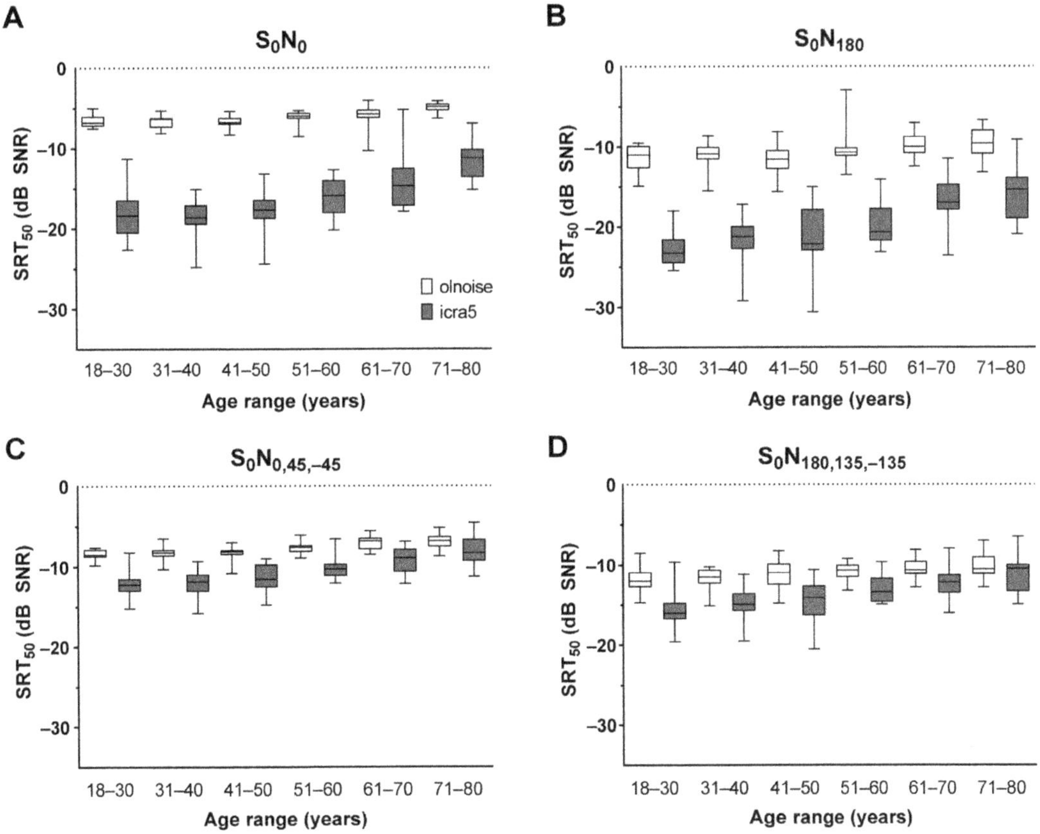

Figure 3. Speech recognition in noise as box plots (median, min, max) for all age groups for the spatial conditions of (**A**) S_0N_0, (**B**) S_0N_{180}, (**C**) $S_0N_{0,45,-45}$, and (**D**) $S_0N_{180,135,-135}$. The SRT_{50} is shown as box plots for the use of olnoise (white) or icra5 noise (grey).

Figure 4 shows the SNR_{cut} distributions for all age distributions, used noise signals and spatial distributions. The specific means and standard deviations are summarised in Table 2. The ANOVA of the SNR_{cut} distribution revealed significant main effects of noise signal (F(1,92) = 266.9, $p < 0.001$), spatial configuration (F(1,92) = 228.2, $p < 0.001$), but not for the between-subjects factor of age group. Only the interaction between noise signal and spatial configuration was significant (F(1,92) = 8.12, $p < 0.01$). The post hoc comparison showed a lower SNR_{cut} for icra5 noise than for olnoise overall and for all spatial configurations. The mean SNR_{cut} was better for the S_0N_{180} presentation compared to the S_0N_0 condition.

Table 3 lists the linear regression results for the variables of age and the binaural PTA. For the S_0N_0 condition with olnoise, a significant linear regression was observed between age and SRT_{50}, and age and SNR_{cut}. The linear regression between age and speech perception in noise was also significant for the $S_0N_{0,45,-45}$ conditions, but not for all other conditions. Binaurally averaged PTA was correlated with speech perception in noise for all conditions except for the S_0N_0 condition. The linear regression between binaural PTA and listening effort in noise was not significant.

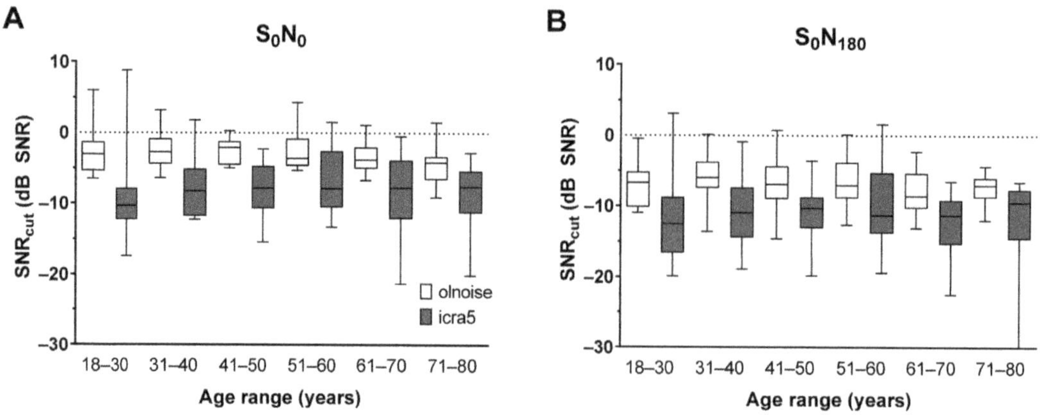

Figure 4. Listening effort in noise as box plots (median, min, max) for all age groups for the spatial conditions of (**A**) S_0N_0 and (**B**) S_0N_{180}. The SNR_{5cut} is shown as box plots for the use of olnoise (white) or icra5 noise (grey).

Table 3. Linear regression report for the outcome variables.

Dependent Variable	Age					PTA, Binaural Average				
Outcome	b	SE	β	T	p	b	SE	β	T	p
Speech perception in noise										
Olnoise, S_0N_0	0.025	0.007	0.438	3.42	**<0.001**	0.013	0.014	0.124	0.97	0.335
Olnoise, S_0N_{180}	0.006	0.015	0.055	0.40	0.689	0.087	0.027	0.441	3.23	**0.002**
Olnoise, $S_0N_{0,45,-45}$	0.018	0.007	3.240	2.74	**0.007**	0.037	0.013	0.348	2.94	**0.004**
Olnoise, $S_0N_{180,135,-135}$	0.010	0.011	0.114	0.88	0.384	0.069	0.021	0.421	3.22	**0.002**
Icra5, S_0N_0	0.035	0.019	0.172	1.89	0.063	0.253	0.035	0.663	7.26	**<0.001**
Icra5, S_0N_{180}	0.031	0.020	0.140	1.49	0.140	0.276	0.038	0.689	7.34	**<0.001**
Icra5, $S_0N_{0,45,-45}$	0.042	0.012	0.341	3.43	**<0.001**	0.109	0.023	0.469	4.70	**<0.001**
Icra5, $S_0N_{180,135,-135}$	0.026	0.015	0.176	1.70	0.093	0.161	0.028	0.591	5.70	**<0.001**
Listening effort in noise										
Olnoise, S_0N_0	−0.044	0.022	−0.301	−2.04	**0.044**	0.026	0.041	0.094	0.64	0.524
Olnoise, S_0N_{180}	−0.031	0.027	−0.175	−1.16	0.248	0.015	0.050	0.045	0.30	0.766
Icra5, S_0N_0	−0.032	0.041	−0.117	−0.78	0.441	0.092	0.076	0.181	1.20	0.232
Icra5, S_0N_{180}	−0.042	0.043	−0.149	−0.98	0.330	0.079	0.080	0.149	0.98	0.331

Bold: significant linear regression, $p < 0.05$.

4. Discussion

The aim of this study was to provide age-related reference signal-to-noise ratios at which 50% speech recognition in noise (SRT_{50}) and moderate listening effort (SNR_{cut}) are assessed by participants. A decline in speech recognition in noise was observed with increasing age. This decrease was significant from the age group of 51–60 years and above. The decrease in SRT_{50} with age was greater when icra5 noise was used than when olnoise was used. Overall, speech could be discriminated at lower SNRs with icra5 noise than with olnoise. Since icra5 allows for listening into gaps in the noise signal ('gap listening' [30]), this finding is consistent with previous results using other speech-modulated noise signals [16,31,32]. For olnoise, the decrease from 18–30 to 71–80 years was smallest for the $S_0N_{0,45,-45}$ condition (1.6 dB) and largest for the $S_0N_{180,135,-135}$ condition (2.12 dB). Using icra5, this difference was also smallest for the $S_0N_{0,45,-45}$ condition (4.46 dB), but largest for the S_0N_0 condition (6.93 dB). The spatial configuration itself also influenced the age-related SRT_{50} and was observed in all age groups. When speech was presented from the front and noise from the back, the best SRT_{50} was observed for both noise signals used. This is consistent with spatial release from masking due to the separation of speech and noise sources [33,34]. However, the measured improvements are still smaller than in a similar study by Decambron et al. [21].

For olnoise, the SRT_{50} was −6.64 dB (SD: 0.75) for the 18–30-year-olds, which is within the range originally reported for the OLSA matrix test [13] and later research [14]. Adding more noise sources improved speech recognition in noise, as the spatial release of masking was increased by adding more correlated noise signal. However, in icra5, the addition of two more noise sources decreased speech intelligibility and thus worsened the SRT_{50}. This finding may be due to the uncorrelated noise signals used in this condition.

Listening effort in noise was influenced by the noise signal used. Speech recognition in icra5 was rated as less demanding, resulting in a lower (better) SNR_{cut} compared to the olnoise conditions. Apparently, the gaps in the speech-modulated noise resulted in better speech recognition, which was rated as less demanding. The presentation of speech and noise from separate sources resulted in less listening effort. No age effect was observed for all spatial and noise conditions.

The observed standard deviations of the SNR_{cut} were larger than those of the SRT_{50}. This may be due to the difficulty of the task. Although the ACALES task was explained in detail, it cannot be excluded that some participants focused more on the speech recognition rating than on the actual listening effort. In such cases, a different internal scale would have been used. The resolution of the scale, with only seven levels, may also have contributed to the larger standard deviation.

Age correlates with increased pure-tone thresholds. It is therefore difficult to disentangle the influence of both factors on speech perception and listening effort in noise. In this study, the influence of the binaurally averaged PTA on both endpoints was assessed by regression analysis. As expected, a correlation between this PTA and the SRT_{50} was observed for most conditions. For the clinically relevant condition of S_0N_0 presentation of noise and speech, this correlation was not significant, but the effect of age was. We conclude that both age and PTA may influence speech perception in noise, at least partially independently. However, the study design, especially the inclusion criteria, has limitations for such an analysis. At younger ages, only participants with good PTA thresholds were included, whereas participants with poorer PTA were only included at older ages. This is reflected in the larger standard deviations and percentiles in the older age groups. This means that younger participants with increased PTA were excluded from the study, which limits a sufficient analysis of the influence of PTA. Also, a specific analysis of high frequency hearing loss, which may correlate with speech-in-noise difficulties, was not performed in this study. Both pure-tone thresholds and age are correlated, but are not the only factors in speech recognition in noise that decline with age. However, many of these factors have to be taken into account when age-related reference values are provided for different age groups.

As speech recognition in noise and listening effort are measured in clinical routines with different spatial configurations and noise signals, this study provides reference data for normal hearing listeners of all ages. The reference values will be useful for comparisons with patient groups such as those with idiopathic sudden hearing loss [35]. In addition to speech recognition in quiet conditions, improved hearing in noise conditions is one of the goals of cochlear implantation and can be used as an indication criterion [36,37]. Especially in patients with unilateral deafness, hearing in noise can be significantly improved by a cochlear implant [38–42] and may be cost-effective compared to no intervention or other interventions [43]. A study of patients with different indications for speech recognition in quiet and noise conditions showed that those patients undergoing cochlear implant candidacy testing who qualified only by a poor hearing in noise had improved hearing in both quiet and noise conditions [44]. As these effects may also be caused by the pre-processing technology in cochlear implants, hearing aid or active middle-ear implant users, different spatial configurations will be required to demonstrate benefits. The age-related reference data reported here may also serve as a benchmark in these cases.

The study results are limited to the German language, as only German-speaking participants were included. In addition, other spatial configurations of speech and noise as well as different noise signals are not covered by the study results. The study did not specifically analyse frequency-specific pure-tone thresholds, which may have differed between age groups.

In conclusion, this study provides reference data on speech perception and listening effort in noise for listeners with age-related hearing loss. In addition to the clinically most relevant spatial condition with frontal speech and noise presentation, this study also provides reference data for more complex spatial conditions and different noise signals.

Author Contributions: Conceptualization, T.R.; Methodology, T.R.; Formal Analysis, T.R. and T.M.W.; Investigation, T.R., A.C.K., L.W. and T.M.W.; Resources, T.R. and S.K.P.; Data Curation, T.R.; Writing—Original Draft Preparation, T.R. and T.M.W.; Writing—Review and Editing, T.R., A.C.K., L.W., T.M.W. and S.K.P.; Visualization, T.R. and T.M.W.; Supervision, T.R.; Project Administration, T.R.; Funding Acquisition, T.R. All authors have read and agreed to the published version of the manuscript.

Funding: This research was funded by Cochlear Research and Development Limited, Addlestone, UK, grant number IIR-2317.

Institutional Review Board Statement: The study was conducted in accordance with the Declaration of Helsinki, and the protocol was approved by the Ethics Committee of the Martin Luther University Halle-Wittenberg (project identification code 2021-044).

Informed Consent Statement: All subjects gave their informed consent for inclusion before they participated in the study.

Data Availability Statement: Supporting raw data may be obtained through special request from the corresponding author.

Acknowledgments: We thank T. Hocke (Cochlear Deutschland GmbH & Co. KG, Hannover, Germany.) for intellectual, administrative, and technical support in designing the experiment.

Conflicts of Interest: T.R. and A.C.K. received funding from Cochlear Research and Development Limited, Addlestone, UK for this work and travel reimbursements. All other authors declare no conflicts of interest. The sponsor had no role in the execution, interpretation, or writing of the study.

References

1. Keithley, E.M. Pathology and mechanisms of cochlear aging. *J. Neurosci. Res.* **2020**, *98*, 1674–1684. [CrossRef]
2. Von Gablenz, P.; Holube, I. Hörverlust und Sprachverstehen im Alter. *Laryngo-Rhino-Otol.* **2017**, *96*, 759–764. [CrossRef]
3. Moore, D.R.; Edmondson-Jones, M.; Dawes, P.; Fortnum, H.; McCormack, A.; Pierzycki, R.H.; Munro, K.J. Relation between speech-in-noise threshold, hearing loss and cognition from 40–69 years of age. *PLoS ONE* **2014**, *9*, e107720. [CrossRef] [PubMed]
4. Lindenberger, U.; Ghisletta, P. Cognitive and sensory declines in old age: Gauging the evidence for a common cause. *Psychol. Aging* **2009**, *24*, 1–16. [CrossRef]
5. Lin, F.R.; Yaffe, K.; Xia, J.; Xue, Q.-L.; Harris, T.B.; Purchase-Helzner, E.; Satterfield, S.; Ayonayon, H.N.; Ferrucci, L.; Simonsick, E.M. Hearing loss and cognitive decline in older adults. *JAMA Intern. Med.* **2013**, *173*, 293–299. [CrossRef] [PubMed]
6. Wingfield, A.; Tun, P.A. Cognitive supports and cognitive constraints on comprehension of spoken language. *J. Am. Acad. Audiol.* **2007**, *18*, 548–558. [CrossRef] [PubMed]
7. Pichora-Fuller, M.K.; Schneider, B.A.; Daneman, M. How young and old adults listen to and remember speech in noise. *J. Acoust. Soc. Am.* **1995**, *97*, 593–608. [CrossRef]
8. Ross, B.; Dobri, S.; Schumann, A. Speech-in-noise understanding in older age: The role of inhibitory cortical responses. *Eur. J. Neurosci.* **2020**, *51*, 891–908. [CrossRef] [PubMed]
9. Kocabay, A.P.; Aslan, F.; Yüce, D.; Turkyilmaz, D. Speech in Noise: Implications of Age, Hearing Loss, and Cognition. *Folia Phoniatr. Logop.* **2022**, *74*, 345–351. [CrossRef]
10. Humes, L.E.; Kidd, G.R.; Lentz, J.J. Auditory and cognitive factors underlying individual differences in aided speech-understanding among older adults. *Front. Syst. Neurosci.* **2013**, *7*, 55. [CrossRef]
11. Füllgrabe, C.; Moore, B.C.J.; Stone, M.A. Age-group differences in speech identification despite matched audiometrically normal hearing: Contributions from auditory temporal processing and cognition. *Front. Aging Neurosci.* **2014**, *6*, 347. [PubMed]
12. Kollmeier, B.; Warzybok, A.; Hochmuth, S.; Zokoll, M.A.; Uslar, V.; Brand, T.; Wagener, K.C. The multilingual matrix test: Principles, applications, and comparison across languages: A review. *Int. J. Audiol.* **2015**, *54* (Suppl. S2), 3–16. [CrossRef] [PubMed]

13. Wagener, K.C.; Brand, T.; Kollmeier, B. Entwicklung und Evaluation eines Satztests für die deutsche Sprache Teil III: Evaluation des Oldenburger Satztests. *Z. Audiol.* **1999**, *38*, 86–95.
14. Abdel-Latif, K.H.A.; Meister, H. Speech Recognition and Listening Effort in Cochlear Implant Recipients and Normal-Hearing Listeners. *Front. Neurosci.* **2021**, *15*, 725412. [CrossRef] [PubMed]
15. Hochmuth, S.; Kollmeier, B.; Brand, T.; Jürgens, T. Influence of noise type on speech reception thresholds across four languages measured with matrix sentence tests. *Int. J. Audiol.* **2015**, *54* (Suppl. S2), 62–70. [CrossRef]
16. Weißgerber, T.; Stöver, T.; Baumann, U. Speech perception in modulated noise assessed in bimodal CI users. *HNO* **2023**, *71*, 487–493. [CrossRef]
17. Chan, D. EUROM—A spoken language resource for the EU. In Proceedings of the 4th European Conference on Speech Communication and Speech Technology Eurospeech, Madrid, Spain, 18–21 September 1995; pp. 867–870.
18. Wagner, F.; Todt, I.; Wagner, J.; Ernst, A. Indications and candidacy for active middle ear implants. *Adv. Oto-Rhino-Laryngol.* **2010**, *69*, 20–26.
19. Puder, H.; Fisher, E.; Hain, J. Optimized Directional Processing in Hearing Aids with Integrated Spatial Noise Reduction. In Proceedings of the IWAENC 2012, International Workshop on Acoustic Signal Enhancement, Aachen, Germany, 4–6 September 2012; VDE Verlag: Offenbach, Germany, 2012.
20. Rahne, T.; Fröhlich, L.; Wagner, L.; Kropp, M.H.; Müller, A. Speech perception and hearing effort using a new active middle ear implant audio processor. *Eur. Arch. Oto-Rhino-Laryngol. Head Neck* **2022**, *279*, 4667–4675. [CrossRef]
21. Decambron, M.; Leclercq, F.; Renard, C.; Vincent, C. Speech audiometry in noise: SNR Loss per age-group in normal hearing subjects. *Eur. Ann. Otorhinolaryngol. Head Neck Dis.* **2022**, *139*, 61–64. [CrossRef]
22. Mukari, S.Z.-M.S.; Wahat, N.H.A.; Mazlan, R. Effects of ageing and hearing thresholds on speech perception in quiet and in noise perceived in different locations. *Korean J. Audiol.* **2014**, *18*, 112–118. [CrossRef]
23. Peelle, J.E. Listening Effort: How the Cognitive Consequences of Acoustic Challenge Are Reflected in Brain and Behavior. *Ear Hear.* **2018**, *39*, 204–214. [CrossRef] [PubMed]
24. Krueger, M.; Schulte, M.; Brand, T.; Holube, I. Development of an adaptive scaling method for subjective listening effort. *J. Acoust. Soc. Am.* **2017**, *141*, 4680. [CrossRef] [PubMed]
25. Kwak, C.; Han, W. Age-Related Difficulty of Listening Effort in Elderly. *Int. J. Environ. Res. Public Health* **2021**, *18*, 8845. [CrossRef]
26. Luts, H.; Eneman, K.; Wouters, J.; Schulte, M.; Vormann, M.; Buechler, M.; Dillier, N.; Houben, R.; Dreschler, W.A.; Froehlich, M.; et al. Multicenter evaluation of signal enhancement algorithms for hearing aids. *J. Acoust. Soc. Am.* **2010**, *127*, 1491–1505. [CrossRef] [PubMed]
27. Magudilu Srishyla Kumar, L. Measuring Listening Effort Using Physiological, Behavioral and Subjective Methods in Normal Hearing Subjects: Effect of Signal to Noise Ratio and Presentation Level. Ph.D. Thesis, James Madison University, Harrisonburg, VA, USA, 2020. Volume 7. Available online: https://commons.lib.jmu.edu/diss202029/7 (accessed on 1 September 2023).
28. Degeest, S.; Keppler, H.; Corthals, P. The Effect of Age on Listening Effort. *J. Speech Lang. Hear. Res.* **2015**, *58*, 1592–1600. [CrossRef]
29. *DIN EN ISO 7029:2017-06*; Akustik- Statistische Verteilung von Hörschwellen in Bezug auf das Alter und das Geschlecht. Beuth Verlag GmbH: Berlin, Germany, 2017.
30. Cooke, M. A glimpsing model of speech perception in noise. *J. Acoust. Soc. Am.* **2006**, *119*, 1562–1573. [CrossRef]
31. Rader, T. Speech Perception of Cochlear Implanted Patients with Combined Electric-Acoustic Stimulation. Ph.D. Thesis, Technische Universität München, Munich, Germany, 2012.
32. Zirn, S.; Polterauer, D.; Keller, S.; Hemmert, W. The effect of fluctuating maskers on speech understanding of high-performing cochlear implant users. *Int. J. Audiol.* **2016**, *55*, 295–304. [CrossRef]
33. Litovsky, R. Spatial release from masking. *Acoust. Today* **2012**, *8*, 18–25. [CrossRef]
34. Wagner, L.; Geiling, L.; Hauth, C.; Hocke, T.; Plontke, S.; Rahne, T. Improved binaural speech reception thresholds through small symmetrical separation of speech and noise. *PLoS ONE* **2020**, *15*, e0236469. [CrossRef]
35. Kitoh, R.; Nishio, S.-Y.; Usami, S.-I. Speech perception in noise in patients with idiopathic sudden hearing loss. *Acta Oto-Laryngol.* **2022**, *142*, 302–307. [CrossRef]
36. Hamzavi, J.; Franz, P.; Baumgartner, W.D.; Gstöettner, W. Hearing performance in noise of cochlear implant patients versus severely-profoundly hearing-impaired patients with hearing aids. *Audiol. Off. Organ Int. Soc. Audiol.* **2001**, *40*, 26–31. [CrossRef] [PubMed]
37. Lundberg, E.M.H.; Strong, D.; Anderson, M.; Kaizer, A.M.; Gubbels, S. Do Patients Benefit from a Cochlear Implant when They Qualify Only in the Presence of Background Noise? *Otol. Neurotol. Off. Publ. Am. Otol. Soc. Am. Neurotol. Soc. Eur. Acad. Otol. Neurotol.* **2021**, *42*, 251–259. [CrossRef] [PubMed]
38. Arndt, S.; Laszig, R.; Aschendorff, A.; Hassepass, F.; Beck, R.; Wesarg, T. Cochlea-Implantat-Versorgung von Patienten mit einseitiger Taubheit oder asymmetrischem Hörverlust. *HNO* **2017**, *65*, 98–108. [CrossRef]
39. Arndt, S.; Wesarg, T.; Stelzig, Y.; Jacob, R.; Illg, A.; Lesinski-Schiedat, A.; Ketterer, M.C.; Aschendorff, A.; Speck, I. Einfluss einseitiger Taubheit auf das Hörvermögen des besseren Ohrs. *HNO* **2020**, *68*, 17–24. [CrossRef] [PubMed]
40. Kitterick, P.T.; Smith, S.N.; Lucas, L. Hearing Instruments for Unilateral Severe-to-Profound Sensorineural Hearing Loss in Adults: A Systematic Review and Meta-Analysis. *Ear Hear.* **2016**, *37*, 495–507. [CrossRef]
41. Rahne, T.; Plontke, S.K. Functional Result After Cochlear Implantation in Children and Adults with Single-sided Deafness. *Otol. Neurotol. Off. Publ. Am. Otol. Soc. Am. Neurotol. Soc. Eur. Acad. Otol. Neurotol.* **2016**, *37*, e332–e340. [CrossRef] [PubMed]

42. Speck, I.; Challier, P.; Wesarg, T.; Jakob, T.F.; Aschendorff, A.; Hassepass, F.; Arndt, S. Is the cochlear implant a successful long-term solution for single-sided deaf and asymmetric hearing-impaired patients. *Eur. Arch. Oto-Rhino-Laryngol.* **2021**, *278*, 3257–3265. [CrossRef]
43. Lee, C.; Yeung, M.W.; Falk, L.; Ali, A.; Walter, M. Implantable Devices for Single-Sided Deafness and Conductive or Mixed Hearing Loss: A Health Technology Assessment. *Ont. Health Technol. Assess. Ser.* **2020**, *20*, 1–165.
44. Mudery, J.A.; Francis, R.; McCrary, H.; Jacob, A. Older Individuals Meeting Medicare Cochlear Implant Candidacy Criteria in Noise but Not in Quiet: Are These Patients Improved by Surgery? *Otol. Neurotol. Off. Publ. Am. Otol. Soc. Am. Neurotol. Soc. Eur. Acad. Otol. Neurotol.* **2017**, *38*, 187–191. [CrossRef]

Journal of
Clinical Medicine

MDPI

Article

Evolving a Model for Cochlear Implant Outcome

Ulrich Hoppe [1,*], Anne Hast [1], Joachim Hornung [1] and Thomas Hocke [2]

1 Cochlear Implant Center CICERO, Department of Otorhinolaryngology-Head and Neck Surgery, Uniklinikum Erlangen, Waldstr. 1, D-91054 Erlangen, Germany; anne.hast@uk-erlangen.de (A.H.); joachim.hornung@uk-erlangen.de (J.H.)

2 Cochlear Deutschland GmbH & Co. KG, Mailänder Str. 4a, D-30539 Hannover, Germany; thocke@cochlear.com

* Correspondence: ulrich.hoppe@uk-erlangen.de; Tel.: +49-(0)9131-8532981

Abstract: Background: Cochlear implantation is an efficient treatment for postlingually deafened adults who do not benefit sufficiently from acoustic amplification. Implantation is indicated when it can be foreseen that speech recognition with a cochlear implant (CI) is superior to that with a hearing aid. Especially for subjects with residual speech recognition, it is desirable to predict CI outcome on the basis of preoperative audiological tests. Purpose: The purpose of the study was to extend and refine a previously developed model for CI outcome prediction for subjects with preoperative word recognition to include subjects with no residual hearing by incorporating additional results of routine examinations. Results: By introducing the duration of unaided hearing loss (DuHL), the median absolute error (MAE) of the prediction was reduced. While for subjects with preoperative speech recognition, the model modification did not change the MAE, for subjects with no residual speech recognition before surgery, the MAE decreased from 23.7% with the previous model to 17.2% with the extended model. Conclusions: Prediction of word recognition with CI is possible within clinically relevant limits. Outcome prediction is particularly important for preoperative counseling and in CI aftercare to support systematic monitoring of CI fitting.

Keywords: word recognition; CI outcome; prediction; generalised linear model; adults

1. Introduction

Cochlear implantation is an efficient treatment for postlingually deafened adults with severe and profound hearing loss. In particular, a cochlear implant (CI) is indicated when the benefit from acoustic amplification is insufficient [1–7]. For mild and moderate hearing loss, a hearing aid (HA) is the option of choice, while for higher degrees of hearing loss, it must be carefully considered which approach is better. Especially in the transition range, i.e., hearing thresholds better than 80 dB_{HL} (dB hearing loss), the variability of the aided speech recognition is substantial [8–17]. Nevertheless, in individual cases the speech recognition with HA can be assessed preoperatively. However, the large variability in CI outcome as assessed by word recognition scores with CI [18–22] represents a major obstacle: for the patient population with benefit from HAs, the *individual* prediction is of major importance, as the patient and the professional have to balance the residual aided word recognition with the HA, the expected word recognition with CI, the expected improvement in quality of life, and the impact of CI surgery. Some studies have also included subjects with lesser hearing loss (e.g., <80 dB_{HL}) who were considered likely to benefit from cochlear implantation [5,6,17,23–29]. A retrospective analysis [22] of 312 postlingually deafened adult CI recipients yielded the preoperative maximum word recognition score (WRS_{max}) as a predictor for the minimum WRS with CI at conversation level, WRS_{65}(CI). The importance of this preoperative measure was confirmed by two studies including, respectively, 128 [28] and 664 [17] cases. In an earlier study we addressed explicitly the prediction of WRS_{65}(CI) in a population with hearing losses of less than 80 dB_{HL} only [6]. This retrospective analysis led to a generalised linear model (GLM) that provides an estimated prediction of $WRS_{65}(CI)$ six months after implantation on the basis of three preoperatively known factors: WRS_{max}, the patient's age at implantation, and the aided WRS at conversation level, $WRS_{65}(HA)$, according to Equation (1).

$$WRS_{65}(CI)[\%] = \frac{100}{1 + e^{-(\beta_0 + \beta_1 \cdot WRS_{max} + \beta_2 \cdot Age + \beta_3 \cdot WRS_{65}(HA))}} \quad (1)$$

with $\beta_0 = 0.84 \pm 0.18$, $\beta_1 = 0.012 \pm 0.0015$, $\beta_2 = -0.0094 \pm 0.0025\ year^{-1}$, and $\beta_3 = 0.0059 \pm 0.0026$; all WRS expressed in %.

Figure 1 illustrates the characteristics of this GLM. WRS_{max} accounts for up to 27 percentage points (pp) in $WRS_{65}(CI)$ differences. $WRS_{65}(HA)$ influences the prediction by up to 9 pp, while age at implantation is associated with a deterioration of up to 17 pp. The GLM resulted from an analysis based on a population of 128 postlingually deafened adult CI recipients, all with a preoperative hearing loss equal to or less than 80 dB_{HL} as measured by the hearing loss at 0.5, 1, 2, and 4 kHz (four-frequency pure-tone average, 4FPTA).

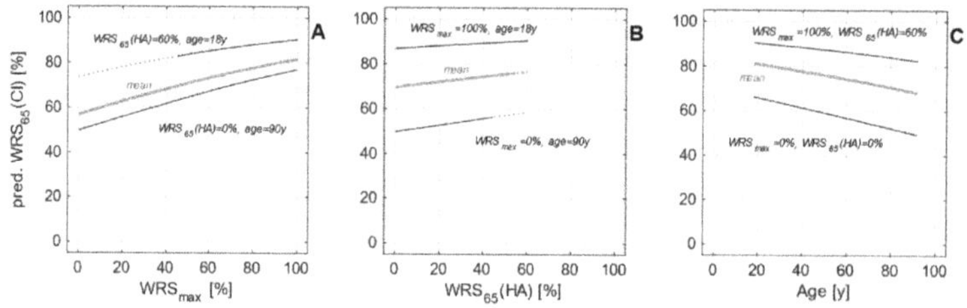

Figure 1. Output characteristics of the generalised linear model as a function of the three input variables within a reasonable input range. The predicted word recognition score $WRS_{65}(CI)$ after six months is shown as a function of (**A**) preoperative maximum word score WRS_{max}, (**B**) preoperative aided score $WRS_{65}(HA)$, and (**C**) age at implantation. In each panel the remaining two factors are kept constant at the selected values indicated, covering the observed range, and the thin black curves show the variation in $WRS_{65}(CI)$. The thick grey curves represent the model's results for the most recent population means at our clinic: WRS_{max} = 50%, $WRS_{65}(HA)$ = 9%, and age = 66 years. Dotted lines indicate a rather unlikely combination of input factors, namely a high $WRS_{65}(HA)$ in the presence of much lower WRS_{max}.

The prediction error of the model as described by the median absolute error (MAE) was found to be 13.5 pp [6], with one-quarter of the study population scoring 12 pp or more below prediction. A subsequent prospective study [29] confirmed the applicability of the model for CI recipients within certain boundary conditions: for a patient population with a preoperative WRS_{max} greater than zero, a prediction error of 11.5 pp was found. Only 6% (5/85) of the recipients missed the predicted score by more than 20 pp within one year after implantation. As shown in Figure 1, the output range is limited to scores between 49% and 90%. This is due to the fact that patients with significant residual hearing are most likely to perform in this range [6,17,22,28,29]. This is not the case for the application of the model in a population with preoperative WRS_{max} = 0%, which, as expected, resulted in a higher prediction error of 23.2 pp. If both WRS_{max} and $WRS_{65}(HA)$ are zero, the prediction from Equation (1) is based solely on the patient's age, represented by β_2, and the population mean outcome, represented by β_0.

While in some previous analyses duration of deafness (DoD) played a significant role [19], DoD was not included in the model (Equation (1)). This is due to the fact that only subjects with hearing threshold better than 80 dB_{HL} were included in the previous study [6]. Holden et al. [20] showed that the duration of hearing impairment (DHI) is a factor that contributes to speech recognition with CI. Additionally, DHI is applicable for subjects with residual hearing, regardless of the degree of hearing loss.

The goal of this study was the extension and evolution of the model [6] in order to improve prediction, especially for patient populations with a preoperative WRS_{max} of zero and all degrees of hearing loss. The design requirements for the model were defined as follows: Since Equation (1) has proved its applicability [29,30], the coefficients $\beta_{0\text{–}3}$ remained fixed. Only preoperative measures were to be included in the model. Additionally, these measures were to be subsets of clinical routine measurements within the CI candidate assessment according to the German CI Guidelines [3] and the German white book CI provision [4].

2. Materials and Methods

2.1. Patients

In this study we evaluated data from all postlingually deafened adult patients who were provided with a Nucleus CI (Cochlear Ltd., Sydney, Australia) in the period April 2020 to December 2022 at the Ear, Nose, and Throat Clinic within the department of Head and Neck Surgery at the University Hospital of Erlangen. All study participants were native German speakers. The CI indication was in accordance with the current German CI guidelines [3]. All participants suffered from sensorineural or mixed hearing loss in the ear to receive the implant. They took part in our rehabilitation programme for a minimum of six months. Rehabilitation was performed in accordance with the most recent recommendations [3,31,32]. Rehabilitation includes speech processor fittings, auditory training, psychological counselling, and medical checks on a regular basis. Usually, rehabilitation is performed for more than twelve months.

Exclusion criterion was cognitive impairment that would have influenced the performance of the speech audiometry. Reimplantations were excluded. Postoperative WRS_{65}(CI) for a period of at least six months after surgery and CI fitting were available for 165 patients. The patient population consisted of 90 men and 75 women. Their mean age at the time of surgery was 66 $\pm$ 14 years. The hearing loss for air conduction was determined as the mean value over the four octave frequencies 0.5, 1, 2, and 4 kHz (4FPTA). For hearing thresholds beyond the maximum possible presentation levels of the audiometers, a value of 130 dB_{HL} was imputed. The resulting mean preoperative hearing loss was 94 $\pm$ 21 dB_{HL}. The 165 CI recipients used either the behind-the-ear processor CP1000 (or later) or the off-the-ear processor CP950 (or later). CI-aided listeners were divided into two groups according to their preoperative WRS_{max}. Group 1 (n = 109) comprised individuals with $WRS_{max} > 0\%$, while group 2 (n = 56) comprised those with $WRS_{max} = 0\%$. While there were no significant differences between these groups in age or in duration of hearing impairment, audiometric data differed owing to the group definitions. Demographic details are summarised in Table 1. Figure 2 complements the characteristics in Table 1 by representing the individual data for age, duration of hearing loss, and duration of unaided hearing loss. Age was not correlated with either duration of hearing impairment (DHI) or duration of unaided hearing impairment (DuHI), while DHI and DuHI were strongly correlated ($R_{Spearman} = 0.68$ with $p = 5 \times 10^{-24}$).

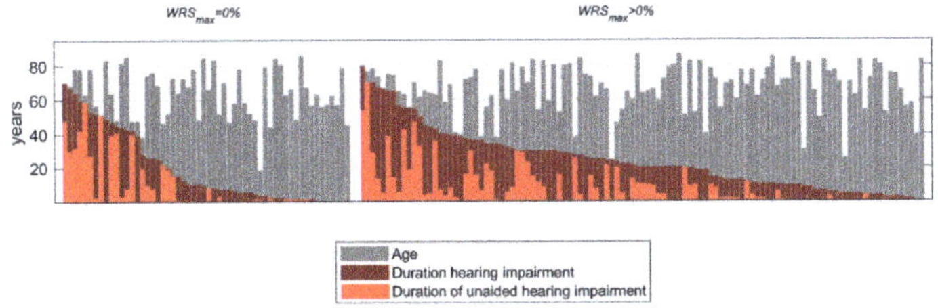

Figure 2. Distribution of age, duration of hearing impairment, and duration of unaided hearing impairment in the two patient groups with preoperative maximum word recognition (WRS_{max}) of zero (**left**) or above zero (**right**).

Table 1. Patient characteristics.

	Size	Age [Years]	4FPTA [dB_{HL}]	WRS_{max} [%]	WRS_{65}(HA)	Duration of Hearing Impairment [Years]	Duration of Unaided Hearing Impairment [Years]	SRT_{num} [dB_{SPL}]
Group 1 $WRS_{max} > 0\%$	109	67 ± 14	83 ± 14	42 ± 23	15 ± 16	24 ± 18	9 ± 13	85 ± 15
Group 2 $WRS_{max} = 0\%$	56	64 ± 14	114 ± 17	0	0 ± 1	20 ± 22	10 ± 16	124 ± 10
total	165	66 ± 14	94 ± 21	27 ± 27	10 ± 15	22 ± 20	9 ± 14	98 ± 23

SRT_{num}, speech recognition threshold for 50% number recognition; SPL, sound pressure level; for other abbreviations, see text above. Means ± standard deviations are shown.

2.2. Speech Audiometry

Speech recognition was assessed by the Freiburg monosyllable and Freiburg two-digit-number tests. The monosyllable test comprises 20 groups of 20 monosyllabic German nouns each; the number test comprises multisyllabic two-digit numbers in 10 groups of 10 numbers each (e.g., 98 was read as "achtundneunzig") [33,34]. Usually, the numbers are understood much better than the monosyllabic words. Recognition rates correspond to low-frequency hearing thresholds [35]. The monosyllable test was used to determine the maximum word recognition score (WRS_{max}), i.e., the word recognition score at the greatest just-tolerable sound pressure level or, in case of 100%, at lower levels. Additionally, WRS_{65}(HA) was defined as the word recognition score with hearing aid measured at 65 dB_{SPL}. The hearing aids were checked technically in advance. In particular, in situ measurements were performed to ensure that the settings yielded the necessary gains [16].

For the Freiburg two-digit numbers, the sound levels were adjusted individually in the range from 30 to 120 dB_{SPL} in 5 dB steps in order to find the sound pressure level for 50% recognition (SRT_{num}). For SRTs above the maximum possible presentation levels of the audiometers, a value of 120 dB_{HL} was imputed. All audiometric measurements were performed monaurally with the ear that was intended for the implant, while the contralateral ear was masked appropriately when necessary.

The 4FPTA was calculated from the pure-tone audiometry data as the mean value of the hearing threshold at 0.5, 1, 2, and 4 kHz.

For the postoperative measurements, the word recognition score with CI system in free field at 65 dB_{SPL}, WRS_{65}(CI) was assessed. The free-field measurements were conducted in a soundproof cabin measuring 6 × 6 m. The loudspeaker was placed 1.5 m in front of the patient (0° azimuth). The contralateral ear was masked appropriately with broadband noise introduced through headphones, if necessary.

2.3. Data Analysis

The software Matlab (MathWorks, Natick, MA, USA) version R2019b was used for all calculations and figures. A GLM was applied to the data to predict WRS_{65}(CI); this model represented a further development of our earlier model (see Section 1) and is described below. Significant differences in word recognition scores were determined according to the characteristics of the Freiburg monosyllable test [36].

3. Results

3.1. Preoperative Measurements

Figure 3A–C show the interrelationships between word recognition scores, WRS_{65}(HA) and WRS_{max}, and the average pure-tone hearing loss, 4FPTA. Figure 3D–F show how speech recognition thresholds for numbers in quiet (SRT_{num}) are related to the 4FPTA and the two WRS. The curves in Figure 3A,B represent WRS as a function of 4FPTA in a population of HA users from previous studies [8,14]. In all cases the preoperative WRS_{65}(HA) was within the current German CI guidelines [3], which recommend a cut-off at 60% for preoperative WRS_{65}(HA). Figure 3D–F illustrate the relationship between the audiometric measures WRS_{65}(HA), WRS_{max}, 4FPTA, and SRT_{num}. Even for cases where WRS_{65}(HA) and WRS_{max} are zero, SRT_{num} can still be measured: there were 95 of 165 cases with WRS_{65}(HA) = 0%, of which 53 (56%) had a measurable SRT_{num}. Among the 56 cases in group 2 (preoperative WRS_{max} = 0%), a measurable SRT_{num} was still found in 12 cases (21%). All speech recognition measures were highly correlated: WRS_{max} with SRT_{num} ($R_{Spearman} = -0.72$ with $p = 6 \times 10^{-28}$), WRS_{65}(HA) with SRT_{num} ($R_{Spearman} = -0.58$ with $p = 2 \times 10^{-16}$), and WRS_{max} with WRS_{65}(HA) ($R_{Spearman} = -0.62$ with $p = 1 \times 10^{-18}$).

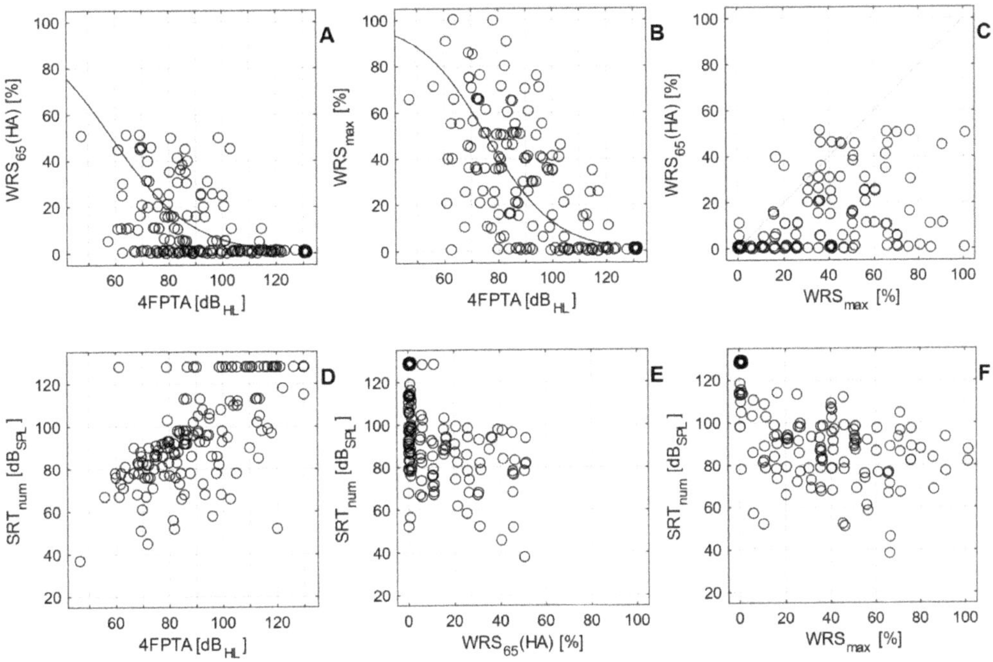

Figure 3. Preoperative audiometry of the 165 cases: (**A**) The aided word recognition score, WRS_{65}(HA), as a function of average pure-tone hearing loss, 4FPTA; (**B**) the maximum word recognition score, WRS_{max}, as a function of 4FPTA; (**C**) relation between WRS_{65}(HA) and WRS_{max}. The black curves in panels (**A**,**B**) represent the average relation between WRS values and 4FPTA in a population of HA users [8,14]. The lower panels (**D**–**F**) show the relationship between SRT_{num} and 4FPTA, WRS_{65}(HA), and WRS_{max}, respectively.

3.2. Postoperative Measurements

Figure 4 illustrates the relationship between the two preoperative WRS and WRS_{65}(CI) six months after surgery. The two groups with WRS_{max} above zero (group 1, black) or equal to zero (group 2, blue) show WRS_{65}(CI) ranging from 0 to 100%. Both groups have their peak in Figure 4C at a WRS_{65}(CI) of 70%, and the median for WRS_{65}(CI) is 70% for both groups. However, the variabilities differed considerably: the standard deviation of WRS_{65}(CI) was 19 pp for group 1 and 30 pp for group 2. Postoperative results are summarised in Table 2.

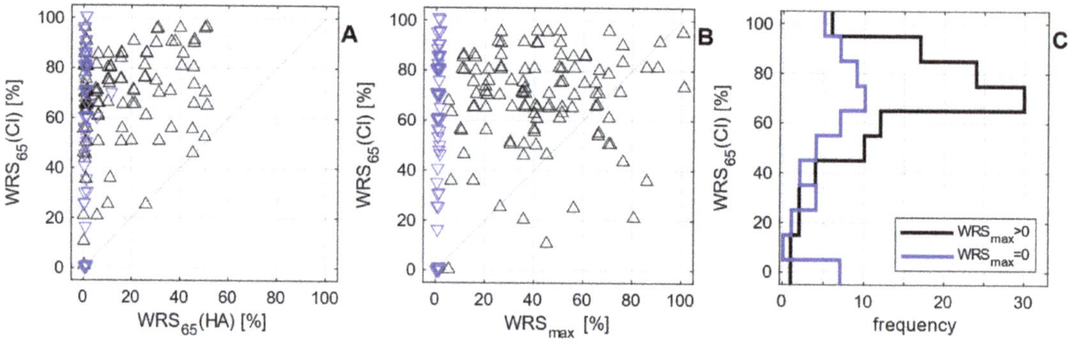

Figure 4. Relationship between preoperative and postoperative word recognition scores for the 165 cases: (**A**) word recognition score with CI after six months (WRS_{65}(CI) vs. the preoperative aided score, WRS_{65}(HA)); (**B**) WRS_{65}(CI) vs. the maximum preoperative word recognition score, WRS_{max}; (**C**) distribution of WRS_{65}(CI) for the two patient groups (black, group 1 with a preoperative WRS_{max} > 0%; blue, group 2 with WRS_{max} = 0%). This colour code applies to panels (**A**,**B**) as well.

Table 2. Variability of word recognition with CI six months after surgery with respect to preoperative maximum word recognition.

Group	Size	WRS_{65}(CI) [%]		No. of Cases with a Score of ...		
		Mean ± SD	Median	WRS_{65}(CI) = 0%	WRS_{65}(CI): >0–<50%	WRS_{65}(CI): 50–100%
Group 1 WRS_{max} > 0%	109	68 ± 19	70	1 (1%)	12 (11%)	96 (88%)
Group 2 WRS_{max} = 0%	56	59 ± 30	70	7 (13%)	9 (16%)	40 (71%)
total	165	65 ± 24	70	8 (5%)	21 (13%)	136 (82%)

With respect to the minimum predictor [22] for WRS_{65}(CI), this study yielded the following results for group 1: Six months after surgery, 6 cases (5.5%) did not reach WRS_{max}, while in 64 cases (58.7%) WRS_{max} was significantly [36] exceeded. The remaining 39 (35.8%) cases reached WRS_{max} within the confidence intervals yielded by the Freiburg test [36].

3.3. Model Expansion

GLMs were applied to the complete data set. As additional input variables to the previous model [6] (see Equation (1)), the duration of hearing impairment (DHI), the duration of unaided hearing impairment (DuHI (a subperiod of DHI)), and SRT_{num} were considered. The strong correlations between SRT_{num} and WRS_{max} and between SRT_{num} and WRS_{65}(HA) (see Section 3.1) indicate that the linear equation system is over-determined.

All regressions with SRT_{num} included resulted in a GLM with a corresponding positive β_i. Such an equation would result in a poorer prediction for WRS_{65}(CI) with better preoperative SRT_{num}. The ablation analysis [37] did not yield an improvement with respect to the overall MAE with SRT_{num} included (12 pp) compared with the final GLM (12 pp). Consequently, the regression analysis was continued with DHI and DuHI only. The ablation analysis yielded the best results applying the two predictors with an interaction term [38]: The overall MAE was 12.3 pp, while for group 1 it was 11.1 pp and for group 2 it was 17.0 pp. Table 3 summarises the results of the regression analysis.

On the basis of Table 3 and with removal of the two non-significant contributors DHI and the interaction term DHI:DuHI, Equation (1) expands to

$$WRS_{65}(CI)[\%] = \frac{100}{1 + e^{-(\beta_0 + \beta_1 \cdot WRS_{max} + \beta_2 \cdot Age + \beta_3 \cdot WRS_{65}(HA) + \beta_0' + \beta_4 \cdot DuHI)}} \quad (2)$$

with $\beta_0 = 0.84 \pm 0.18$, $\beta_1 = 0.012 \pm 0.0015$, $\beta_2 = -0.0094 \pm 0.0025$ year^{-1}, $\beta_3 = 0.0059 \pm 0.0026$, $\beta_0' = 0.35 \pm 0.04$, and $\beta_4 = -0.0171 \pm 0.0056$ year^{-1} (all WRS expressed in %), as shown in Table 3.

Table 3. Results of regression analysis with two additional predicting variables and their interaction term, duration of hearing impairment (DHI), and duration of unaided hearing impairment (DuHI). The coefficients from the previous model [6] were fixed.

	Estimate	Standard Error	t Statistic	p
Constant, β_0'.	0.35	0.04	8.44	3×10^{-17}
DHI [year^{-1}]	−0.0027	0.0019	−1.41	0.16
DuHI, β_4 [year^{-1}]	−0.0171	0.0056	−3.05	0.002
DHI:DuHI [year^{-2}]	−4.20	0.0001	−0.41	0.68

Included are 6600 observations, 6596 error degrees of freedom. χ^2 statistic vs. constant model: 152, $p = 1 \times 10^{-32}$.

The application of Equation (2) to the study population yields prediction errors as shown in Figure 5, separately for the two groups. A comparison with the previous model [6] is displayed as well.

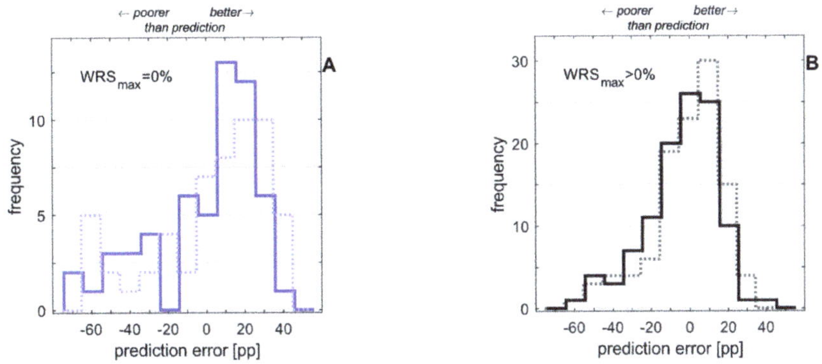

Figure 5. Distribution of differences between predicted and measured word recognition with CI and WRS_{65}(CI), six months after surgery: (**A**) prediction errors in percentage points (pp) for group 1 (preoperative $WRS_{max} > 0$); (**B**) prediction errors for group 2 ($WRS_{max} = 0$). In both panels the dotted line indicates the prediction error resulting from the application of the previous model [6] (Equation (1)). The solid line indicates the prediction error resulting from the advanced model (Table 3). The MAE was 11.1 pp in group 1 and 17.1 pp in group 2 according to Equation (2). The previous model resulted in MAEs of 11.3 pp for group 1 and 23.7 pp for group 2.

In cases where DuHI is not available in the clinical data set, a regression analysis with DHI would be helpful. Consequently, this was done. Table 4 summarises the results of this analysis. On the basis of Table 4, Equation (1) expands to

$$\mathrm{WRS}_{65}(\mathrm{CI})[\%] = \frac{100}{1 + e^{-(\beta_0 + \beta_1 \cdot \mathrm{WRS}_{\max} + \beta_2 \cdot \mathrm{Age} + \beta_3 \cdot \mathrm{WRS}_{65}(\mathrm{HA}) + \beta_0' + \beta_4 \cdot \mathrm{DHI})}} \quad (3)$$

with $\beta_0 = 0.84 \pm 0.18$, $\beta_1 = 0.012 \pm 0.0015$, $\beta_2 = -0.0094 \pm 0.0025$ year^{-1}, $\beta_3 = 0.0059 \pm 0.0026$, $\beta_0' = 0.41 \pm 0.04$, and $\beta_4 = -0.0125 \pm 0.0013$ year^{-1} (all WRSs expressed in %), as shown in Table 4.

Table 4. Results of regression analysis with one additional predicting variable only: duration of hearing impairment (DHI). The coefficients from the previous model [6] were fixed.

	Estimate	Standard Error	t Statistic	p
Constant, β_0'.	0.41	0.04	10.75	6×10^{-27}
DHI, β_4 [year^{-1}]	−0.0125	0.0013	−9.73	2×10^{-22}

Included are 6600 observations, 6598 error degrees of freedom. χ^2-statistic vs. constant model: 96.4, $p = 1 \times 10^{-22}$.

The resulting MAEs are 11.3 pp for group 1 and 18.8 pp for group 2, with an overall MAE of 14.0 pp.

4. Discussion

The vast majority (89%) of the patients included in this study showed signifearimproved speech recognition without any patient experiencing a lower WRS six months after cochlear implantation.

Both populations (patients with preoperative WRS_{max} larger than zero, group 1, and patients with preoperative WRS_{max} equal to zero, group 2) showed a median WRS_{65}(CI) of 70%. However, as illustrated by Figure 4, the variability of the outcome was greater for group 2, and the mean WRS_{65}(CI) was smaller: 59% in group 2, compared with 68% in group 1. Additionally, group 2 includes seven subjects (13%) with WRS_{65}(CI) = 0, while in group 1, only one subject (1%) scored 0%. These subjects clearly indicate the demand for future studies dealing with unexpected low speech perception.

The extension of the prediction model for CI outcome in CI recipients with preoperative $WRS_{max} = 0$ is feasible. It was shown that for group 2 an improved prediction is possible without impairment of the prediction for group 1. Most remarkably, the inclusion of just one additional input variable (the duration of unaided hearing impairment, DuHI) in the previous prediction model for the WRS_{65}(CI) [6] resulted in a decreased prediction error for group 2: the new GLM (Equation (2)) resulted in a decreased MAE of 17.0, compared with the MAE of the previous model (Equation (1)) of 23.7 pp. The prediction error for group 1 remained almost unchanged: the new model indicates a slightly decreased MAE of 11.1 pp, compared with 11.4 obtained from the previous model [6].

The results demonstrate that it is possible to use one model for both groups. This enables a seamless application for all CI candidates independently from the preoperative speech recognition. It may be used as a baseline for further refinements of the model for specific candidate groups. However, this would require by far a greater number of cases. The durations of hearing impairment and unaided hearing impairment, DHI and DuHI, were found to be strongly correlated ($R_{Spearman} = 0.7$). Hence, they may provide similar information on the CI outcome. The ablation analysis showed that the MAE was not greatly increased when DHI or DuHI was omitted. We decided to retain the latter because DHI was found as not significant ($p = 0.16$) in the presence of DuHI. Additionally, the MAE was smaller for both groups when DuHI was used instead of DHI (Equation (2)). However, the DHI offers some advantages. The DHI is just defined by one time point, the time of onset of hearing loss, while determination of DuHI requires knowledge of two time points: HA provision and onset of hearing loss. Yet both factors depend on the patient's ability to remember or reconstruct events which may well have occurred decades earlier. In summary, the model according to Equation (3) inherits larger MAE. However, Equation (3) and therefore the DHI may be used in cases where DuHI is not available.

In this study, the DHI replaces the previously used duration of deafness, DoD. Though DoD was frequently used in CI studies, it is not well defined; regarding DoD, an obsolete classification [39] refers to a cut-off of 81 dB_{HL} for the grade "profound impairment including deafness". A more recent classification from WHO [40] defines "Complete or total hearing loss/deafness" as hearing threshold in the better ear of 95 dB_{HL} or greater. Those authors explicitly explain that the PTA should not be used as the "sole determinant for rehabilitation" and that "the classification and grades are for epidemiological use" [40].

For prediction models and clinical process management, to our knowledge, there is a lack of applicable, defined criteria for cut-off relating to the duration of deafness and hearing impairment. Additionally, in the presence of a decentralised hearing health care system (e.g., in Germany), the chance of obtaining all necessary data retrospectively is rather low. In our population of consecutive Nucleus CI provisions in adults within a period of 2.5 years, the majority is not deaf using this definition, so a broader application of DoD in a regression model is not relevant. In addition, about one-third of the patients defined as "deaf" using the above WHO criterion [40] had a measurable ipsilateral maximum recognition score for Freiburg words, and slightly under one-half had a measurable speech recognition threshold for Freiburg numbers in quiet. This supports the preference for functional, speech-related variables instead of DoD.

There was a slight decrease in MAE for group 1 only (preoperative $WRS_{max} > 0$). This can be interpreted as giving strong support to the use of WRS_{max} for predictive purposes [6,17,22,28], as it accumulates the detrimental effects of long DHI (or DuHI). The situation is different in group 2 (preoperative $WRS_{max} = 0$), where such functional assessment with the established test WRS_{max} and WRS_{65}(HA) is not possible. Here, the additional information of DuHI or DHI considerably reduces the prediction error.

According to the design requirements, the regression analysis using the GLM was conducted across all data by using all data in a first attempt. The effects of these three variables upon the prediction error are different. It was found that SRT_{num} did not decrease MAE. Hence, SRT_{num} was not taken into account any longer, which however does not necessarily mean that this variable is unimportant. Together with the strong correlation with WRS_{max} and WRS_{65}(HA), this indicates an over-determined equation system. Nevertheless, especially for cases with no preoperative monosyllable speech perception, it might be a useful addition. In our population only about one-quarter of group 2 had a measurable SRT_{num}. Perhaps an additional split beyond groups 1 and 2 will improve the prediction with the help of SRT_{num} in a clearly and more narrowly defined population. On the other hand, other model approaches—such as random forest regression—would induce such a split per se. However, more data would be needed for such an approach. In a recent study, Rieck et al. [17] used the Freiburg numbers and found a predictive value in a population of nearly 500 recipients. Two characteristics of their study population would support the assertion of a positive impact of SRT_{num} on prediction error in a population with low preoperative speech perception in general. The mean values obtained in their study represent the characteristics of an established patient population with a preoperative mean WRS_{65}(HA) of 4.2% compared with 9.7% and a WRS_{max} of 11.8 compared with 27.6% in this population. Rieck et al. [17] included clinical data with implantations dating from 2002 to 2019, while the inclusion period of the present study was from 2020 to 2022. Consequently, this relationship should be reconsidered in future studies that include more CI candidates who are in group 2 but who have measurable SRT_{num}.

5. Conclusions

Cochlear implantation can be considered if speech recognition with hearing aids is insufficient. This applies also for patients with pure-tone hearing loss in the range of 60 dB_{HL}. The preoperative prediction of expected word recognition after CI provision is possible within clinically relevant limits.

Less variable results for postoperative word recognition were observed in patients with preoperative maximum word recognition greater than zero (group 1) compared with patients without preoperative maximum word recognition (group 2).

The inclusion of additional model input variables—'duration of hearing impairment' or 'duration of unaided hearing impairment'—to the variables 'word recognition scores' and 'age at implantation' already used in the model resulted in decreased prediction errors for group 2. However, the prediction error in group 2 was still larger than in group 1. In group 1 the inclusion of additional input variables did not result in a lower prediction error.

We believe that this model will be applicable in preoperative counseling (with a higher accuracy in group 1 than in group 2) and will also be useful in CI aftercare to support the systematic monitoring of CI fitting that is conducted to optimise postoperative adjustment.

Author Contributions: Conceptualisation, U.H. and J.H.; methodology, U.H.; software, T.H. and U.H.; validation, A.H. and J.H.; writing—original draft preparation, U.H. and T.H.; writing—review and editing, U.H. and A.H.; visualization, T.H.; supervision, J.H. All authors have read and agreed to the published version of the manuscript.

Funding: This research was partially funded by Cochlear Research & Development Ltd. (IIR2398).

Institutional Review Board Statement: The study was conducted in accordance with the Declaration of Helsinki and approved by the Institutional Review Board of Erlangen University, No. 60_20B 6 March 2020.

Informed Consent Statement: Informed consent was obtained from all subjects involved in the study.

Data Availability Statement: Research data are available on request from the first author.

Conflicts of Interest: T.H. is working for a cochlear implant company. All other authors declare no conflict of interest. The funders had no role in the design of the study, in the data collection or in the decision to publish the results.

References

1. National Institute for Health and Care Excellence. Cochlear Implants for Children and Adults with Severe to Profound Deafness. 2019. Available online: https://www.nice.org.uk/guidance/ta566 (accessed on 1 June 2023).
2. Buchman, C.A.; Gifford, R.H.; Haynes, D.S.; Lenarz, T.; O'Donoghue, G.; Adunka, O.; Biever, A.; Briggs, R.J.; Carlson, M.L.; Dai, P.; et al. Unilateral Cochlear Implants for Severe, Profound, or Moderate Sloping to Profound Bilateral Sensorineural Hearing Loss: A Systematic Review and Consensus Statements. *JAMA Otolaryngol. Head Neck Surg.* **2020**, *146*, 942–953. [CrossRef] [PubMed]
3. AWMF. Leitlinien: Cochlea-Implantat Versorgung und Zentral-Auditorische Implantate. 2020. Available online: https://www.awmf.org/uploads/tx_szleitlinien/017-071l_S2k_Cochlea-Implantat-Versorgung-zentral-auditorische-Implantate_2020-12.pdf (accessed on 1 June 2023).
4. DGHNO-KHC. Weißbuch Cochlea-Implantat(CI)-Versorgung. 2nd Edition. 2021. Available online: https://cdn.hno.org/media/2021/ci-weissbuch-20-inkl-anlagen-datenblocke-und-zeitpunkte-datenerhebung-mit-logo-05-05-21.pdf (accessed on 1 June 2023).
5. Van der Straaten, T.F.K.; Briaire, J.J.; Vickers, D.; Boermans, P.; Frijns, J.H.M. Selection Criteria for Cochlear Implantation in the United Kingdom and Flanders: Toward a Less Restrictive Standard. *Ear Hear.* **2020**, *42*, 68–75. [CrossRef]
6. Hoppe, U.; Hocke, T.; Hast, A.; Iro, H. Cochlear Implantation in Candidates with Moderate-to-Severe Hearing Loss and Poor Speech Perception. *Laryngoscope* **2021**, *131*, E940–E945. [CrossRef] [PubMed]
7. Turton, L.; Souza, P.; Thibodeau, L.; Hickson, L.; Gifford, R.; Bird, J.; Stropahl, M.; Gailey, L.; Fulton, B.; Scarinci, N.; et al. Guidelines for Best Practice in the Audiological Management of Adults with Severe and Profound Hearing Loss. *Semin. Hear.* **2020**, *41*, 141–246. [CrossRef] [PubMed]
8. Hoppe, U.; Hast, A.; Hocke, T. Audiometry-Based Screening Procedure for Cochlear Implant Candidacy. *Otol. Neurotol.* **2015**, *36*, 1001–1005. [CrossRef]
9. McRackan, T.R.; Fabie, J.E.; Burton, J.A.; Munawar, S.; Holcomb, M.A.; Dubno, J.R. Earphone and Aided Word Recognition Differences in Cochlear Implant Candidates. *Otol. Neurotol.* **2018**, *39*, e543–e549. [CrossRef]
10. Kronlachner, M.; Baumann, U.; Stover, T.; Weissgerber, T. Investigation of the quality of hearing aid provision in seniors considering cognitive functions. *Laryngorhinootologie* **2018**, *97*, 852–859. [CrossRef]
11. Franks, Z.G.; Jacob, A. The speech perception gap in cochlear implant patients. *Cochlear Implants Int.* **2019**, *20*, 176–181. [CrossRef]
12. Lupo, J.E.; Biever, A.; Kelsall, D.C. Comprehensive hearing aid assessment in adults with bilateral severe-profound sensorineural hearing loss who present for Cochlear implant evaluation. *Am. J. Otolaryngol.* **2020**, *41*, 102300. [CrossRef]
13. Weissgerber, T.; Muller, C.; Stover, T.; Baumann, U. Speech perception and cognitive abilities in seniors without subjective hearing loss. *Laryngorhinootologie* **2019**, *98*, 489–496. [CrossRef]
14. Dörfler, C.; Hocke, T.; Hast, A.; Hoppe, U. Speech recognition with hearing aids for 10 standard audiograms. *HNO* **2020**, *68*, 93–99. [CrossRef] [PubMed]
15. Digeser, F.M.; Engler, M.; Hoppe, U. Comparison of bimodal benefit for the use of DSL v5.0 and NAL-NL2 in cochlear implant listeners. *Int. J. Audiol.* **2020**, *59*, 383–391. [CrossRef] [PubMed]
16. Engler, M.; Digeser, F.; Hoppe, U. Effectiveness of hearing aid provision for severe hearing loss. *HNO* **2022**, *70*, 520–532. [CrossRef]
17. Rieck, J.H.; Beyer, A.; Mewes, A.; Caliebe, A.; Hey, M. Extended Preoperative Audiometry for Outcome Prediction and Risk Analysis in Patients Receiving Cochlear Implants. *J. Clin. Med.* **2023**, *12*, 3262. [CrossRef] [PubMed]

18. Krüger, B.; Joseph, G.; Rost, U.; Strauss-Schier, A.; Lenarz, T.; Büchner, A. Performance groups in adult cochlear implant users: Speech perception results from 1984 until today. *Otol. Neurotol.* **2008**, *29*, 509–512. [CrossRef]
19. Blamey, P.J.; Artieres, F.; Baskent, D.; Bergeron, F.; Beynon, A.; Burke, E.; Dillier, N.; Dowell, R.; Fraysse, B.; Gallégo, S.; et al. Factors affecting auditory performance of postlinguistically deaf adults using cochlear implants: An update with 2251 patients. *Audiol. Neurotol.* **2013**, *18*, 36–47. [CrossRef] [PubMed]
20. Holden, L.K.; Finley, C.C.; Firszt, J.B.; Holden, T.A.; Brenner, C.; Potts, L.G.; Gotter, B.D.; Vanderhoof, S.S.; Mispagel, K.; Heydebrand, G.; et al. Factors affecting open-set word recognition in adults with cochlear implants. *Ear Hear.* **2013**, *34*, 342–360. [CrossRef] [PubMed]
21. Zeh, R.; Baumann, U. Inpatient rehabilitation of adult CI users: Results in dependency of duration of deafness, CI experience and age. *HNO* **2015**, *63*, 557–576. [CrossRef]
22. Hoppe, U.; Hocke, T.; Hast, A.; Iro, H. Maximum preimplantation monosyllabic score as predictor of cochlear implant outcome. *HNO* **2019**, *67*, 62–68. [CrossRef]
23. Helbig, S.; Adel, Y.; Rader, T.; Stover, T.; Baumann, U. Long-term Hearing Preservation Outcomes After Cochlear Implantation for Electric-Acoustic Stimulation. *Otol. Neurotol.* **2016**, *37*, e353–e359. [CrossRef]
24. Dalbert, A.; Huber, A.; Baumann, N.; Veraguth, D.; Roosli, C.; Pfiffner, F. Hearing Preservation After Cochlear Implantation May Improve Long-term Word Perception in the Electric-only Condition. *Otol. Neurotol.* **2016**, *37*, 1314–1319. [CrossRef] [PubMed]
25. Buchman, C.A.; Herzog, J.A.; McJunkin, J.L.; Wick, C.C.; Durakovic, N.; Firszt, J.B.; Kallogjeri, D. Assessment of Speech Understanding After Cochlear Implantation in Adult Hearing Aid Users: A Nonrandomized Controlled Trial. *JAMA Otolaryngol. Head Neck Surg.* **2020**, *146*, 916–924. [CrossRef] [PubMed]
26. Kelsall, D.; Lupo, J.; Biever, A. Longitudinal outcomes of cochlear implantation and bimodal hearing in a large group of adults: A multicenter clinical study. *Am. J. Otolaryngol.* **2021**, *42*, 102773. [CrossRef]
27. Walia, A.; Shew, M.A.; Kallogjeri, D.; Wick, C.C.; Durakovic, N.; Lefler, S.M.; Ortmann, A.J.; Herzog, J.A.; Buchman, C.A. Electrocochleography and cognition are important predictors of speech perception outcomes in noise for cochlear implant recipients. *Sci. Rep.* **2022**, *12*, 3083. [CrossRef]
28. Thangavelu, K.; Nitzge, M.; Weiß, R.M.; Mueller-Mazzotta, J.; Stuck, B.A.; Reimann, K. Role of cochlear reserve in adults with cochlear implants following post-lingual hearing loss. *Eur. Arch. Oto-Rhino-Laryngol.* **2022**, *280*, 1063–1071. [CrossRef]
29. Hoppe, U.; Hast, A.; Hocke, T. Validation of a predictive model for speech discrimination after cochlear implant provision. *HNO* **2023**, *71*, 53–59. [CrossRef] [PubMed]
30. Dziemba, O.C.; Merz, S.; Hocke, T. Evaluative audiometry after cochlear implant provision. *HNO* **2023**. [CrossRef]
31. Dazert, S.; Thomas, J.P.; Loth, A.; Zahnert, T.; Stöver, T. Cochlear implantation—Diagnosis, indications, and auditory rehabilitation results. *Dtsch. Arztebl. Int.* **2020**, *117*, 690–700. [CrossRef]
32. Stöver, T.; Plontke, S.K.; Guntinas-Lichius, O.; Welkoborsky, H.J.; Zahnert, T.; Delank, K.W.; Deitmer, T.; Esser, D.; Dietz, A.; Wienke, A.; et al. Conception and implementation of a certification system for quality control of cochlear implant treatment in Germany. *HNO* **2023**, *71*, 73–81. [CrossRef]
33. Hahlbrock, K.H. *Sprachaudiometrie: Grundlagen und Praktische Anwendung Einer Sprachaudiometrie für das Deutsche Sprachgebiet*; Thieme Verlag: Stuttgart, Germany, 1957.
34. *DIN45621-1:1995-08*; Word Lists for Recognition Tests–Part 1: Monosyllabic and Polysyllabic Words. Beuth Berlin: Berlin, Germany, 1995.
35. Braun, T.; Wimmer, M.; Hempel, J.M. Two formulas for exact calculation of hearing loss for numbers. *HNO* **2012**, *60*, 814–816. [CrossRef]
36. Winkler, A.; Holube, I. Test-retest reliability of the Freiburg monosyllabic speech test. *HNO* **2016**, *64*, 564–571. [CrossRef] [PubMed]
37. Cohen, P.R.; Howe, A.E. How Evaluation Guides AI Research: The Message Still Counts More Than the Medium. *AI Mag.* **1985**, *9*, 35–43. [CrossRef]
38. Matlab Documentation. 2023. Available online: https://de.mathworks.com/help/stats/wilkinson-notation.html (accessed on 12 June 2023).
39. Olusanya, B.O.; Davis, A.C.; Hoffman, H.J. Hearing loss grades and the International classification of functioning, disability and health. *Bull. World Health Organ.* **2019**, *97*, 725–728. [CrossRef] [PubMed]
40. World Health Organization. *World Report on Hearing*; World Health Organization: Geneva, Switzerland, 2021. Available online: https://www.who.int/publications/i/item/9789240020481 (accessed on 12 June 2023).

Journal of
Clinical Medicine

MDPI

Article

Factors to Describe the Outcome Characteristics of a CI Recipient

Matthias Hey [1,*], Kevyn Kogel [1], Jan Dambon [1], Alexander Mewes [1], Tim Jürgens [2] and Thomas Hocke [3]

[1] ENT Clinic, UKSH Kiel, 24105 Kiel, Germany; kevyn.kogel@uksh.de (K.K.); janandreas.dambon@uksh.de (J.D.); stu226070@mail.uni-kiel.de (A.M.)
[2] Institute of Acoustics, University of Applied Sciences Lübeck, 23562 Lübeck, Germany; tim.juergens@th-luebeck.de
[3] Cochlear Deutschland, 30539 Hannover, Germany; thocke@cochlear.com
* Correspondence: hey@audio.uni-kiel.de; Tel.: +49-431-500-21857

Abstract: Background: In cochlear implant (CI) treatment, there is a large variability in outcome. The aim of our study was to identify the independent audiometric measures that are most directly relevant for describing this variability in outcome characteristics of CI recipients. An extended audiometric test battery was used with selected adult patients in order to characterize the full range of CI outcomes. **Methods**: CI users were recruited for this study on the basis of their postoperative results and divided into three groups: low (1st quartile), moderate (medium decentile), and high hearing performance (4th quartile). Speech recognition was measured in quiet by using (i) monosyllabic words (40–80 dB SPL), (ii) speech reception threshold (SRT) for numbers, and (iii) the German matrix test in noise. In order to reconstruct demanding everyday listening situations in the clinic, the temporal characteristics of the background noise and the spatial arrangements of the signal sources were varied for tests in noise. In addition, a survey was conducted using the Speech, Spatial, and Qualities (SSQ) questionnaire and the Listening Effort (LE) questionnaire. **Results**: Fifteen subjects per group were examined (total N = 45), who did not differ significantly in terms of age, time after CI surgery, or CI use behavior. The groups differed mainly in the results of speech audiometry. For speech recognition, significant differences were found between the three groups for the monosyllabic tests in quiet and for the sentences in stationary (S0°N0°) and fluctuating (S0°NCI) noise. Word comprehension and sentence comprehension in quiet were both strongly correlated with the SRT in noise. This observation was also confirmed by a factor analysis. No significant differences were found between the three groups for the SSQ questionnaire and the LE questionnaire results. The results of the factor analysis indicate that speech recognition in noise provides information highly comparable to information from speech intelligibility in quiet. **Conclusions**: The factor analysis highlighted three components describing the postoperative outcome of CI patients. These were (i) the audiometrically measured supra-threshold speech recognition and (ii) near-threshold audibility, as well as (iii) the subjective assessment of the relationship to real life as determined by the questionnaires. These parameters appear well suited to setting up a framework for a test battery to assess CI outcomes.

Keywords: cochlear implant; speech recognition; signal processing; speech audiometry

1. Introduction

Cochlear implants (CIs) represent an option for patients with profound hearing loss [1–3] or with insufficient residual speech recognition [4,5] and today, in some countries, even for asymmetrical hearing loss of various degrees [6].

At the very beginning of CI provision, the observed postoperative word recognition scores (WRS) were rather low because most patients had long-standing and high-degree hearing loss before the implantation [7]. CI candidacy has changed from the beginning of clinical cochlear implant care [2,7–10] to nowadays, where the vast majority of CI recipients show improved speech perception after CI provision [11–16], as up to two-thirds of the patients have a preoperative residual speech recognition [17,18].

As soon as larger populations were investigated, the enigma of (unexplained) poor performance [19,20] became evident, and it still persists [17,18]. Several attempts have been made to identify predictive factors for WRS after CI provision [12,14,19,21,22]. Those studies focussed on the relationships between various preoperative and postoperative measurements in order to predict the results of the latter ones. Supra-threshold presentation of monosyllabic words at 65 dB in quiet was mainly considered [14,19,21,23].

For the postoperative assessment of implantable hearing systems, a large number of measures may be feasible [4,24–26]. Supra-threshold measures of monosyllabic words at the conversational presentation level are widely used [12,19,21,24]. Everyday listening situations include speech in quiet as well in noise [27–29]. Recent data logging studies with speech processors indicate that low-level speech is also present to a substantial extent [30–32]. Audiometric surrogate parameters for low-level speech include word or sentence recognition scores at 40 and/or 50 dB SPL and speech reception thresholds (SRT) of numbers [24,33–36].

An aspect that has more recently been a focus in speech audiometry research is the increased focus on ecological validity. As a result, tests using sentences in noise are nowadays also obligatory in aftercare [6]. Matrix tests using different spatial loudspeaker configurations and competing signal conditions are in wide use [37–40].

Complementing the audiometric assessment, patient-reported outcome measures have become an established tool in the aftercare of recipients of implanted hearing systems. Numerous questionnaires, visual analog scales, and ecological momentary assessments [41,42] are available. These have been adapted to the special requirements of patients with hearing systems.

The availability of so many audiological methods raises the question of which ones should be chosen for use in routine clinical audiometry. Together, all these measures represent a statistically overdetermined system, an assertion that is supported by the many correlations found among the various outcome measures [24,43,44]. Two aspects are worth considering in view of such overdetermination: (i) the burden of time and concentration for the patient limits the daily available time frame; (ii) clinical resources should be allocated with maximum efficiency.

The aim of this study was to identify the most relevant measures, specifically those that provide information independent of other measures, for the purpose of describing as completely as possible the outcome characteristics of CI recipients. It was not the aim of this study to investigate the causes of the poor performance, but to describe the reliable audiological assessment of this performance with regard to the available methods.

Therefore, a test battery based on Hoth and Müller-Deile [24] was extended to measure numerous different outcome parameters in CI patients. The test battery consisted of speech recognition in quiet for numbers and the performance intensity function of words in quiet, which are known to provide useful information for postoperative rehabilitation, system fitting [24,34,36,45], and its considerable importance for everyday life as derived from data logging studies [28,32]. Furthermore, sentences in quiet, sentences in noise with different kinds of noise and different loudspeaker configurations, and questionnaires for subjective patient feedback on speech recognition, directional hearing, hearing quality, and listening effort were included in the test battery.

This test battery was investigated with patients representing the whole range of best, moderately, and poorly performing patients, following the classification proposed by Rieck et al. [23]. An exploratory principal component analysis (PCA) was used to investigate the variability within the three groups with respect to this test battery. Since the portion of poorly performing patients is relatively low [11,18,21,46] to allow for a PCA, all poor-performing subjects had to be included. Afterward, the resulting group size was matched by the moderately and best-performing groups.

2. Materials and Methods

2.1. Research Participants and Classification

Forty-five participants were recruited for this study, which was approved and conducted in accordance with local university ethics approval (study ID 444/23; 23 February 2023). All procedures involving human participants were performed in accordance with the ethical standards of the institutional and national research committee, as well as the 1964 Helsinki Declaration and its later amendments or comparable ethical standards.

All patients were adults with post-lingual onset of deafness. They had received Nucleus cochlear implants (Cochlear Limited, Macquarie Park, NSW, Australia) and had been using them for at least one year [12,47,48]. They were recruited from our clinical database, which included 538 individuals [23].

The patients were classified on the basis of their performance in the Freiburg monosyllabic test at 70 dB SPL conducted two years (instead of one case at 1 year) after receiving the CIs.

Those who scored above the third quartile were considered to have good speech recognition performance and were termed 'high performers' (HP). Patients who scored below the first quartile were termed 'low performers' (LP). Patients in the median range (45th to 55th percentile) were referred to as 'moderate performers' (MP). The classification was performed monaurally and excluded patients who received binaural treatment with different outcome levels (one side HP and one side LP) as well as CI recipients with normal hearing in the other ear.

2.2. Audiometric Test Procedures

The tests were conducted in a sound-shielded audiometric test booth [49] using calibrated loudspeakers placed 1 m away from the patient. Participants with bilateral or bimodal hearing were tested on one ear with the contralateral sound processor switched off and the non-tested ear masked if necessary. If both ears were in the same performance group, patients were allowed to choose which ear to use.

All speech comprehension tests were presented through a computer-based audiometer (Equinox; Interacoustics, Middelfart, Denmark with evidENT 3 software, Merz Medizintechnik, Reutlingen, Germany). For speech in quiet, the Freiburg monosyllabic words were applied frontally [50] at presentation levels of 40, 50, 65, and 80 dB SPL. Items from each list were presented in randomized order to minimize any repetitive learning effect. Additionally, the SRT for Freiburg two-digit numbers was measured. The "percent correct" score of a measured list of 10 numbers (greater or smaller than 50%) was used to increase or decrease the presentation level in 5 dB steps for the subsequent list. The SRT was determined by interpolation.

For speech recognition in noise, the Oldenburg sentences (a German version of a Matrix test) were used [37], containing 30 sentences for each list. An adaptive procedure [51] was applied aiming to determine the SRT (the signal-to-noise ratio (SNR) yielding a 50% words correct score). All of the CI users in this study were accustomed to this adaptive test procedure. To reduce the procedural learning effect with the Oldenburg sentence test [52], training was conducted (one list of 30 sentences) before each session. Afterward, the words correct score for the Oldenburg sentences in quiet was measured at 70 dB SPL using 30 sentences. For investigation in noise, according to Hey et al. [52], only recipients with an SRT in S_0N_0 (speech and stationary Oldenburg noise from front) better than 5 dB SNR were included. If a patient was unable to meet this criterion, the SRT was set to 5 dB SNR for further analysis. In addition to this measurement, which is the widely used quasi-standard for measurements in noise [53,54], we used a setup aiming for more ecological validity. This implemented the Oldenburg sentences with fluctuating Icra5 noise [55] and separated signal sources: speech coming from the front and the competing signal coming from the side of the CI (S_0N_{CI}) [56].

2.3. Questionnaires

To obtain individual subjective feedback on the sound quality obtained with the CI sound processors, the German version of the SSQ questionnaire [57,58] was used, which is known to show a high test–retest accuracy [59]. Additionally, the listening effort questionnaire [60] was used on the same day as speech testing.

Hearing quality in the patients' everyday lives was determined by using the short version of the German SSQ questionnaire [58]. This questionnaire contains a total of 17 items for the categories of speech recognition, directional hearing, and hearing quality. The rating scale for the SSQ questionnaire items ranges from not at all (0) to perfect (10). A high scale value corresponds to a good assessment of the corresponding hearing situation.

To rate the listening effort of CI patients, the questionnaire of Schulte et al. [58] was chosen. This questionnaire focuses on the categories 'understanding in noise', 'understanding with impaired signal quality', and 'understanding in quiet and with lip-reading', with a total of 17 questions. It shows results on a rating scale ranging from not stressful (0) to extremely stressful (10); thus, a high scale value corresponds to a poor assessment of the corresponding hearing situation.

2.4. Analysis

Data are presented as boxplots. Each boxplot shows the median (solid center line), the 25th and 75th percentiles (box limits), and the 5th and 95th percentiles (whiskers) on the left, with individual scores indicated on the right. The Kruskal–Wallis test was used for group comparison. Subsequent post hoc analyses were carried out using the Wilcoxon rank sum test.

The PCA was carried out using the maximum likelihood method. The analysis of the data using the multivariate Henze–Zirkler test for normal distribution showed that a multivariate normal distribution can be assumed, which is a prerequisite for this analysis method [61]. Analysis was performed using Matlab (Mathworks Inc., Natick, MA, USA). If a patient was unable to perform the sentence test adequately in stationary noise, this SRT was set to +5 dB SNR in order to take account of missing data [52]. A comparable procedure was used for the sentence test in fluctuating background noise, where the SRT was set to 10 dB SNR if a value was missing.

3. Results

A total of 45 CI patients were recruited for the study. They were assigned to three groups: LP, MP, and HP. The study measurements for speech audiometry in quiet and the questionnaires were successfully completed for all users examined except one LP subject who did not do the questionnaire. Table 1 provides further information about the participants. The mean age of the subjects in the LP group was noticeably lower than in the HP and MP groups, and the mean time since CI implantation was shorter in the MP group than in the HP and LP groups. The usage time of CIs differs only slightly between the groups. However, these differences for age, time after CI surgery, and usage time of CI per day were not statistically significant (Kruskal–Wallis test; $\chi^2 = 5.14$, $p = 0.08$; $\chi^2 = 0.85$, 0.66 and $\chi^2 = 0.82$, $p = 0.66$, respectively) and are not considered likely to have influenced the study's result.

Table 1. Patient details. For age, duration of fitting, and use time per day, mean values and standard deviations are given. The side in hearing solution characterizes the tested ear. Groups are assigned as follows: LP—low performer, MP—moderate performer, and HP—low performer.

	Study Population	LP Group	MP Group	HP Group
Group Size	**45**	**15**	**15**	**15**
Age (years)	61.4 ± 12.6	55.7 ± 12.9	63.7 ± 14.0	64.8 ± 9.3
Time after CI surgery (years)	6.2 ± 4.1	7.0 ± 5.3	4.8 ± 1.6	6.9 ± 4.3
Use time of CI per day (h)	13.7 ± 3.0	13.0 ± 3.7	13.4 ± 2.5	14.7 ± 2.7
Hearing solution				
binaural (right)	14	4	5	5
binaural (left)	9	4	1	4
bimodal (right)	14	5	5	4
bimodal (left)	4	0	2	2
monaural (right)	2	1	1	0
monaural (left)	2	1	1	0
Speech processor				
CP1100	2	1	0	1
CP1000	37	13	13	11
CP1000 Hybrid	2	0	0	2
CP910	3	1	2	0
CP910 Hybrid	1	0	0	1
Cochlear implant				
CIx32	33	9	14	10
CIx12	4	2	0	2
CI24RE(CA)	8	4	1	3

The results for speech recognition for the Freiburg WRS are shown as box plots depending on stimulation level for the three patient groups examined in Figure 1. The grouping of the patients was based on postoperative speech recognition with CIs [23]. All patients confirmed their allocation to the LP, MP, and HP groups in the Freiburg word test [62] according to its test–retest accuracy. Patients of the low-performing group showed higher variability in speech test data, as the first quartile of the performance includes monosyllabic words correct score from 0% up to 55%.

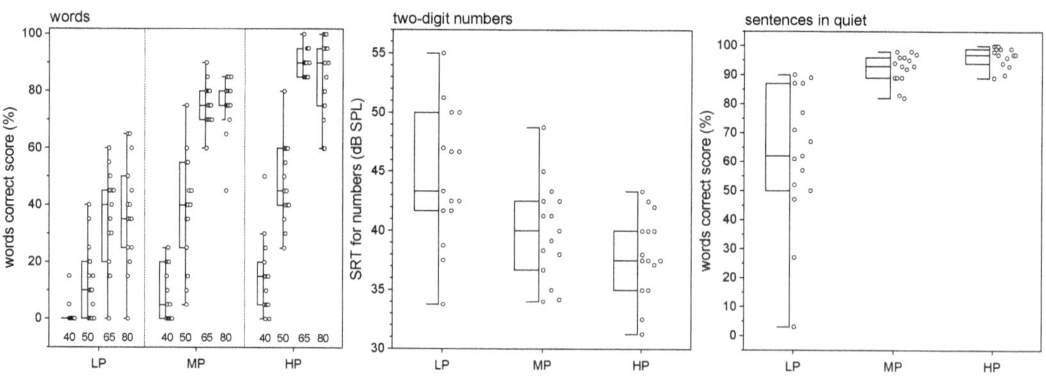

Figure 1. Speech recognition in quiet is presented as boxplots. (**Left**) Grouped data of words correct score for Freiburg monosyllabic words depending on presentation level. (**Middle**) SRT for two-digit numbers. (**Right**) Words correct score for Oldenburg sentences. Groups are assigned as follows: LP—low performer, MP—moderate performer, and HP—high performer.

For a presentation level of 80 dB SPL, the median speech recognition was 90% for the HP group, 75% for the MP group, and 35% for the LP group. The Kruskal–Wallis test revealed significant differences between the groups, as confirmed by the Wilcoxon rank sum test in a post hoc analysis for HP–LP ($p < 0.001$, zvalue = 4.45) and MP–LP ($p < 0.001$, zvalue = −4.44) pairs and, less clearly significant, HP–MP ($p = 0.03$, zvalue = 2.12). At 65 dB SPL, the median speech recognition for the HP, MP, and LP groups was 90%, 75%, and 40%, respectively. Significant differences between the groups were also found at this level with the Kruskal–Wallis test, and the Wilcoxon rank sum test confirmed these differences between all groups with $p < 0.001$ (HP-LP zvalue = 4.68, HP-MP zvalue = 4.23, MP-LP = −4.65). At 50 dB SPL, the Kruskal–Wallis test also showed significant differences between the groups, which were confirmed by the Wilcoxon rank sum test between HP and LP ($p < 0.001$, zvalue = 4.36) and MP and LP ($p < 0.001$, zvalue = −3.46); however, the HP and MP groups ($p = 0.16$, zvalue = 1.42) did not differ significantly at this SPL level. The measurement results at 40 dB SPL showed significant differences in speech recognition between the three groups. However, the post hoc analysis showed a significant difference only between HP and LP ($p < 0.001$, zvalue = 3.83).

The results of the SRT for Freiburg numbers are shown in Figure 1 (middle). The Kruskal–Wallis test confirms a significant difference between the three groups ($\chi^2 = 11.11$, $p < 0.01$) and the following post hoc analysis HP–LP ($p < 0.01$, zvalue = −3.12) and MP–LP ($p = 0.03$, zvalue = 2.22).

The results of the Oldenburg sentences in quiet are shown in Figure 1 on the right. The Kruskal–Wallis test showed that there were significant differences between the three groups.

Figure 2 (left) shows the results of the SRT for the Oldenburg sentences in stationary noise and frontal presentation of speech and noise as boxplots. The median SRT for the HP group was −2.8 dB SNR, with a range of 0.25 to −5.45 dB SNR. Figure 2 (right), in contrast, shows speech recognition in fluctuating noise with spatially separated signal sources. The HP and MP groups revealed no significant difference ($p = 0.06$, zvalue = −1.85).

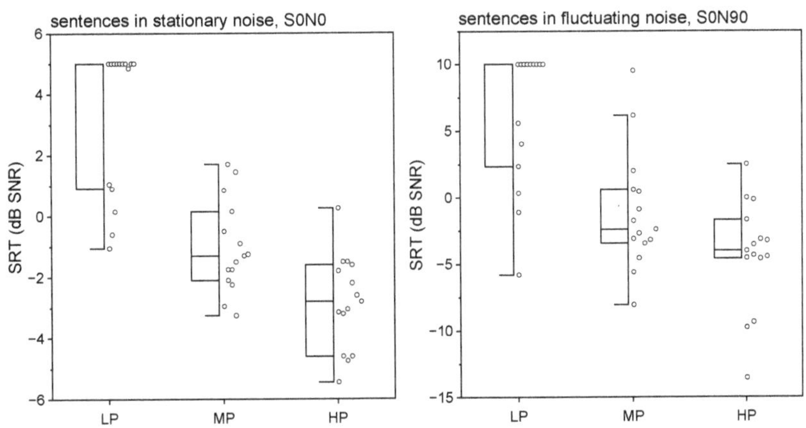

Figure 2. Speech recognition in noise presented as boxplots. (**Left**) SRT for the Oldenburg sentences in stationary noise; speech and noise from the front. (**Right**) SRT for the Oldenburg sentences in fluctuating noise; speech from the front and noise from the side of the CI.

The results of the patients' subjective feedback using two questionnaires are shown in Figure 3. No significant differences were found between the performance groups. It should be added that the performance groups did not differ significantly in the SSQ subdomains (Kruskal–Wallis for speech understanding $\chi^2 = 3.3$; $p = 0.20$, for spatial orientation $\chi^2 = 2.8$; $p = 0.25$, listening quality $\chi^2 = 3.3$; $p = 0.19$, and listening effort $\chi^2 = 5.3$; $p = 0.07$).

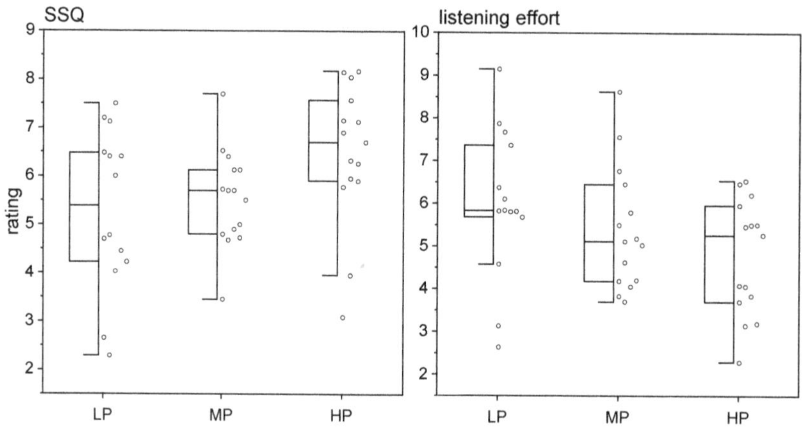

Figure 3. Results of the questionnaires for the three sub-groups as boxplots. (**Left**) SSQ questionnaire. A high SSQ value corresponds to a positive evaluation for the situations surveyed. (**Right**) Listening effort questionnaire. A high value on the listening effort questionnaire scale corresponds to a negative evaluation for the situations surveyed.

A PCA was carried out using the maximum likelihood method. The analysis of the data with the multivariate Henze–Zirkler test for normal distribution showed that a multivariate normal distribution ($p = 0.21$, HZ lognormal variance = 0.02, HZ statistic = 0.98) can be assumed, which is a prerequisite for this analysis method [61]. The Kaiser–Meyer–Olkin measure for determining the intercorrelation between the variables was 0.87. According to Klopp [61], this corresponds to a good suitability of the data for a factor analysis. The results of the factor analysis are shown in Table 2. The analysis of the eigenvalues revealed that no more than three factors should be selected for calculation, as the eigenvalue for the fourth factor is clearly below one at 0.51. This indicates that most of the observed variances can be well explained by the first three factors. Analysis of the eigenvalues showed that 84% of the variability is explained by the first three components, with 60% for the 1st, 14% for the 2nd, and 10% for the 3rd component.

Table 2. PCA after Varimax rotation for data from speech audiometry and questionnaires. Bold numbers indicate relevance for a given factor.

	1st Component	2nd Component	3rd Component
SRT for numbers	−0.24	**−0.75**	−0.17
Words 40 dB SPL	0.22	**0.68**	0.05
Words 50 dB SPL	0.47	**0.86**	0.05
Words 65 dB SPL	**0.82**	0.45	0.20
Words 80 dB SPL	**0.88**	0.26	0.25
Sentences in quiet	**0.81**	0.32	0.27
SRT in stationary noise (S0N0)	**−0.79**	−0.41	−0.19
SRT in fluctuating noise (S0NCI)	**−0.81**	−0.22	−0.13
Questionnaire 'SSQ'	0.14	0.10	**0.98**
Questionnaire 'listening effort'	−0.21	−0.07	**−0.53**

Results for supra-threshold speech audiometry (WRS at 65 and 80 dB SPL, sentences in quiet as well as in stationary and fluctuating noise) show high absolute value loadings on factor 1, with the highest value for monosyllabic words at 80 dB SPL. Near-threshold speech tests (numbers, words at 40 and 50 dB SPL) are dominant for the 2nd factor. The questionnaires show a clear loading for the 3rd factor; this applies in particular to the SSQ.

4. Discussion

In our investigation, we measured audiometric and subjective outcome parameters for a group of 45 experienced CI patients. To address the issue of poor performance, we weighted the share of poor performers equally with the shares of excellent and medium performers, allowing reliable differentiation between those groups.

The basic audiometric characteristics of a CI recipient can be described by three main components: (1) *Supra-threshold speech recognition*, (2) near-threshold *audibility*, and the subjectively perceived benefit referred to as (3) *patient-reported outcome*. Most remarkably, speech recognition in noise did not load a separate component but was the same as supra-threshold speech recognition in quiet.

All patients in the HP and MP groups were able to perform all audiometric and subjective outcome tests of the complete test battery, unlike some patients in the LP group, in which nine persons were unable to perform the two sentences tests in noise. Their correct score in noise was too low to allow the performance of the adaptive procedure [52]. However, responses for patient-reported outcome measures and 'numbers in quiet' were adequate, as all patients were able to respond. For monosyllabic words at different test levels, the measurement procedure could be performed for all patients, although some of the recipients showed a score of 'no words correct'. Nevertheless, for this test, it was an adequate measure in the LP group, and this result corresponds well with the overall performance of such recipients, as has also been described elsewhere [18].

Browning et al. [63] stated that good speech comprehension can be achieved in different ways. The way in which this is achieved is not the focus of the present study, which primarily concerns an adequate description of the outcome in relation to speech recognition, which is the main goal of CI therapy for high degrees of hearing loss.

According to the Kaiser–Meyer–Olkin value of 0.86, the data collection of this test battery provides a good basis for PCA and the further interpretation presented here.

4.1. 1st Component—Supra-Threshold Speech Recognition

The following considerations arise in the interpretation: The first component is described by supra-threshold comprehension. This applies to word comprehension at 65 and 80 dB SPL as well as to the sentence tests in quiet and in noise, which were also carried out at a presentation level of 65 dB SPL. The highest loading of the first component was observed for the monosyllabic word test at 65 and 80 dB SPL and sentences in quiet and noise at 65 dB SPL. On the basis of the present findings and the other investigations [64,65], we would have expected a separate component for comprehension in noise. Surprisingly, to account for variability, speech recognition in noise does load on the same component as conversational level speech in quiet. Weissgerber et al. [46] found that age is the only predicting factor for SRT in noise in a selected group of CI patients with a preoperative maximum WRS greater than 0%. In the present study, the three groups did not differ significantly in age. This may explain the fact that speech in noise did not contribute additional information in our PCA.

4.2. 2nd Component—Audibility

Instead of speech recognition in noise, the second component is loaded by monosyllabic WRSs and multisyllabic numbers at lower levels of speech at 50 dB SPL and below. This can be interpreted as audibility [34,45]. The highest representation in this second component is WRS at 50 dB SPL. However, we would recommend the SRT for numbers or an equivalent measure, as this is free of floor effects, while the WRS at low stimulation level yielded in a very large portion of the LP a value of 0%. Additionally, the assessment of the SRT is less frustrating for the CI users while still yielding the information contained in the 2nd component. Furthermore, the numbers are highly redundant. Consequently, the number test represents more audibility and less lexical effects than the monosyllabic test material. The correlation between all near-threshold scores should not be misinterpreted as an argument for omitting assessment of the discrimination function: in this study, we included patients who, in our opinion, were well aided (fitted) [24]. They had completed postoperative rehabilitation and showed stable fitting of their speech processor. However, in order to identify any fitting issues, a mismatch between scores at different levels within the discrimination function of monosyllables can give valuable hints for optimizing the speech processor settings [24,34,36]. Additionally, WRS at medium and even low levels is important for everyday communication [32].

4.3. 3rd Component—Patient-Reported Outcome

The third component is loaded by the patient's perspective on everyday life as assessed by questionnaires. This component is loaded most strongly by SSQ and to a much lesser degree by listening effort. For the German AWMF guideline [53], this is taken into account by the recommended use of the Nijmegen Cochlear Implantation Questionnaire (NCIQ) [66]. The 3rd component can be considered a valuable addition in postoperative quality assurance. Patient-reported outcome measures represent an important part of the outcome measure, but one cannot completely determine the outcome by questionnaires. It has to be mentioned that audiometric measures are not a reliable predictor of patient-reported outcomes in CI patients [67]. On the other hand, audiometric measures of performance prior to CI surgery do not show a reliable correlation to postoperative quality-of-life scores [68]. In the 3rd component, the three groups are hardly distinguishable (see below and in the paragraph Limitations).

Nevertheless, the measure explains the additional variability of 10%. The different preoperative baselines of the individual recipients may provide a rationale for this finding. It is reasonable to assume that a recipient with poor preoperative audiological condition may perceive a great subjective benefit even if his/her WRS is poor compared with that of other recipients [69]. Consequently, the smaller share of variability explained by the third component should not be misinterpreted as implying that subjective rating is only of low importance.

4.4. Limitations of the Study

Study participants were grouped according to their former WRS, as this score is the audiometric hub for all therapeutic decisions according to the AWMF guidelines. Consequently, this measure loads the 1st component strongly.

A limited set of audiometric procedures was applied in this study. There is a variety of other German-language tests, such as the following tests in quiet and in noise: the Sotscheck test, the Göttingen and HSM sentences tests, and the digit-triplet test. Furthermore, more spatial settings—as used in recent studies [13,35,40,70]—were not included here. The subset of possible audiometric tests was selected by consideration of the limited time available for concentrated testing of the patients.

The present study did not analyze objective procedures such as electrode impedances, or electrophysiological [71], anatomical [11], and mapping parameters [34,36,45,64]. The focus here was not on fitting but on describing independent determinants of outcome. These additional variables provide the basis for the subject of further, currently ongoing studies.

The selection of patients for this study was based on speech recognition as the dominant target parameter, as described in the AWMF guidelines [53] and various earlier studies [12,19,72]. The audiometric test procedures used separated the LP, MP, and HP groups well. However, this separation was not recognized for patient-reported outcome measures. This may have been due to the fact that other aspects are tested here. For example, the listening effort for HP patients can be high, as they may be integrated into a normal acoustic listening environment through their occupation and are exposed to more background noise than LP patients.

There are also other approaches for defining poor performance in characterizing CI outcomes. In the present study, absolute postoperative performance was used. Another way would have been to consider postoperative performance in comparison with preoperative auditory status—i.e., relative performance, as described by Hoppe et al. [18,23], according to whom specifications for poor performance are hard to meet because they apply to only very few patients of the total collective.

However, the aim here was not to describe the treatment of the LP but only to characterize it. This tool can now be used for patient collectives at other centers and with different CI systems. This test battery might be used for further evaluation of poor-performing patients. This topic of cases with unexpectedly poor speech perception was motivated by Moberly [20] and was described in more detail with respect to speech recognition by Hoppe et al. [18].

5. Conclusions

Within the outcome-measure framework for CI patients used here in relation to the specific research or clinical question, a proposal for a test battery for evaluating the therapeutic success of a CI was developed. The three components of audiometrically measured supra-threshold comprehension and audibility, as well as subjective rating of relationship to real life through the questionnaires, are well suited for such a framework.

Results of the study suggest the use of (i) monosyllabic words at 65 and/or 80 dB SPL, (ii) monosyllabic words at 50 dB SPL and/or SRT of numbers, and (iii) the SSQ questionnaire as a minimum test inventory.

Author Contributions: Conceptualization, M.H.; methodology, all authors; software, K.K. and J.D.; validation, M.H. and T.J.; formal analysis, K.K. and M.H.; investigation, K.K. and J.D.; resources, M.H.; data curation, K.K. and J.D.; writing—original draft preparation, M.H. and T.H.; writing—review and editing, all authors; visualization, K.K. and M.H.; supervision, M.H.; project administration, K.K.; funding acquisition, M.H. All authors have read and agreed to the published version of the manuscript.

Funding: This study was supported by Cochlear Europe Ltd. (IIR 2193).

Institutional Review Board Statement: This Study was approved and conducted in accordance with CAU University Kiel ethics approval (study ID 444/23 on 23 February 2023).

Informed Consent Statement: Informed consent was obtained from all subjects involved in the study prior to the investigation.

Data Availability Statement: Data are provided within the manuscript.

Acknowledgments: We cordially thank all the patients who kindly took the time to participate in the investigation.

Conflicts of Interest: Thomas Hocke is an employee of Cochlear Deutschland GmbH & Co KG. The remaining authors declare that the research was conducted in the absence of any commercial or financial relationships that could be construed as a potential conflict of interest. The authors alone are responsible for the content and writing of this paper.

References

1. Clark, G. (Ed.) *Cochlear Implants. Fundamentals and Applications*; Springer: New York, NY, USA, 2003. [CrossRef]
2. Lehnhardt, E.; Battmer, R.D.; Nakahodo, K.; Laszig, R. Cochlear implants. *HNO* **1986**, *34*, 271–279. [PubMed]
3. Dhanasingh, A.; Hochmair, I. Thirty Years of Translational Research Behind MED-EL. *Acta Oto-Laryngol.* **2021**, *141*. [CrossRef] [PubMed]
4. NICE. Cochlear implants for children and adults with severe to profound deafness. *NICE Technol. Apprais. Guid.* **2019**, *166*, 1–41.
5. Van Der Straaten, T.F.K.; Briaire, J.J.; Vickers, D.; Boermans, P.P.B.M.; Frijns, J.H.M. Selection Criteria for Cochlear Implantation in the United Kingdom and Flanders: Toward a Less Restrictive Standard. *Ear Hear.* **2021**, *42*, 68–75. [CrossRef]

6. Lailach, S.; Neudert, M.; Zahnert, T. Update Cochlea-Implantation: Indikationsstellung und Operation. *Laryngo-Rhino-Otol.* **2021**, *100*, 652–672. [CrossRef]
7. Laszig, R.; Lehnhardt, E. Cochlear implant. Ein elektronische Hörprothese. *Dt. Ärztebl.* **1987**, *45*, 3033–3038.
8. Battmer, R.D.; Lehnhardt, E. Clark implantable auditory prosthesis. Prerequisites and technic; report on the cochlear implant project of the ENT clinic of the Medical School in Hannover. *Fortschritte Der Med.* **1985**, *103*, 397–400.
9. Battmer, R.D.; Lehnhardt, E.; Laszig, R. The promontory test and electrocochleography with reference to indications for cochlear implant. *HNO* **1986**, *34*, 139–142.
10. Burian, K.; Hochmair-Desoyer, I.J.; Eisenwort, B. The Vienna cochlear implant program. *Otolaryngol. Clin. N. Am.* **1986**, *19*, 313–328. [CrossRef]
11. Franke-Trieger, A.; Lailach, S.; Shetty, J.; Murrmann, K.; Zahnert, T.; Neudert, M. Word Recognition with a Cochlear Implant in Relation to Prediction and Electrode Position. *J. Clin. Med.* **2023**, *13*, 183. [CrossRef]
12. Holden, L.K.; Finley, C.C.; Firszt, J.B.; Holden, T.A.; Brenner, C.; Potts, L.G.; Gotter, B.D.; Vanderhoof, S.S.; Mispagel, K.; Heydebrand, G.; et al. Factors affecting open-set word recognition in adults with cochlear implants. *Ear Hear.* **2013**, *34*, 342–360. [CrossRef] [PubMed]
13. Büchner, A.; Schwebs, M.; Lenarz, T. Speech understanding and listening effort in cochlear implant users—Microphone beamformers lead to significant improvements in noisy environments. *Cochlear Implant. Int.* **2020**, *21*, 1–8. [CrossRef] [PubMed]
14. Thangavelu, K.; Nitzge, M.; Weiß, R.M.; Mueller-Mazzotta, J.; Stuck, B.A.; Reimann, K. Role of cochlear reserve in adults with cochlear implants following post-lingual hearing loss. *Eur. Arch. Oto-Rhino-Laryngol.* **2022**, *280*, 1063–1071. [CrossRef] [PubMed]
15. Rauch, A.K.; Metzner, T.; Aschendorff, A.; Arndt, S.; Speck, I.; Laszig, R.; Beck, R.L. Speech processor upgrade increases speech comprehension in patients with cochlear implants. *Hno* **2019**, *67*, 778–785. [CrossRef] [PubMed]
16. Wimmer, W.; Weder, S.; Caversaccio, M.; Kompis, M. Speech intelligibility in noise with a pinna effect imitating cochlear implant processor. *Otol. Neurotol.* **2016**, *37*, 19–23. [CrossRef]
17. Beyer, A.; Rieck, J.-H.; Mewes, A.; Dambon, J.A.; Hey, M. Erweiterte präoperative sprachaudiometrische Diagnostik im Rahmen der Cochleaimplantatversorgung. *HNO* **2023**, *71*, 779–786. [CrossRef] [PubMed]
18. Hoppe, U.; Hast, A.; Hornung, J.; Hocke, T. Evolving a Model for Cochlear Implant Outcome. *J. Clin. Med.* **2023**, *12*, 6215. [CrossRef]
19. Blamey, P.; Artieres, F.; Başkent, D.; Bergeron, F.; Beynon, A.; Burke, E.; Dillier, N.; Dowell, R.; Fraysse, B.; Gallégo, S.; et al. Factors affecting auditory performance of postlinguistically deaf adults using cochlear implants: An update with 2251 patients. *Audiol. Neurotol.* **2012**, *18*, 36–47. [CrossRef] [PubMed]
20. Moberly, A.C.; Bates, C.; Harris, M.S.; Pisoni, D.B. The Enigma of Poor Performance by Adults With Cochlear Implants. *Otol. Neurotol.* **2016**, *37*, 1522–1528. [CrossRef]
21. Hoppe, U.; Hocke, T.; Hast, A.; Iro, H. Cochlear Implantation in Candidates with Moderate-to-Severe Hearing Loss and Poor Speech Perception. *Laryngoscope* **2021**, *131*, E940–E945. [CrossRef]
22. Goudey, B.; Plant, K.; Kiral, I.; Jimeno-Yepes, A.; Swan, A.; Gambhir, M.; Büchner, A.; Kludt, E.; Eikelboom, R.H.; Sucher, C.; et al. A MultiCenter Analysis of Factors Associated with Hearing Outcome for 2735 Adults with Cochlear Implants. *Trends Hear.* **2021**, *25*. [CrossRef]
23. Rieck, J.H.; Beyer, A.; Mewes, A.; Caliebe, A.; Hey, M. Extended Preoperative Audiometry for Outcome Prediction and Risk Analysis in Patients Receiving Cochlear Implants. *J. Clin. Med.* **2023**, *12*, 3262. [CrossRef] [PubMed]
24. Hoth, S.; Müller-Deile, J. Audiologische Rehabilitation von Kochleaimplantat-Trägern. *HNO* **2009**, *57*, 635–648. [CrossRef] [PubMed]
25. Maier, H.; Baumann, U.; Baumgartner, W.-D.; Beutner, D.; Caversaccio, M.D.; Keintzel, T.; Kompis, M.; Lenarz, T.; Magele, A.; Mewes, T.; et al. Minimal Reporting Standards for Active Middle Ear Hearing Implants. *Audiol. Neurotol.* **2018**, *23*, 105–115. [CrossRef]
26. Beutner, D.; Adano; Delb, W.; Frenzel, H.; Hoppe, U.; Hüttenbrink, K.B.; Mlynski, R.; Limberger, A.; Schönweiler, R.; Schwab, B.; et al. Guideline "Implantable hearing aids"—Short version: German S2k guideline of the Working Group of German-speaking Audiologists, Neurootologists and Otologists (ADANO), of the German Society of Oto-Rhino-Laryngology, Head and Neck Surgery (DGHNO) in collabo. *HNO* **2018**, *66*, 654–659. [CrossRef] [PubMed]
27. Busch, T.; Vanpoucke, F.; van Wieringen, A. Auditory environment across the life span of cochlear implant users: Insights from data logging. *J. Speech Lang. Hear. Res.* **2017**, *60*, 1362–1377. [CrossRef]
28. Oberhoffner, T.; Hoppe, U.; Hey, M.; Hecker, D.; Bagus, H.; Voigt, P.; Schicktanz, S.; Braun, A.; Hocke, T. Multicentric analysis of the use behavior of cochlear implant users. *Laryngo-Rhino-Otol.* **2018**, *97*, 313–320. [CrossRef]
29. Hey, M.; Hocke, T.; Ambrosch, P. Speech audiometry and data logging in CI patients: Implications for adequate test levels. *HNO* **2018**, *66*, S22–S27. [CrossRef]
30. Wu, Y.H.; Stangl, E.; Zhang, X.; Bentler, R.A. Construct validity of the ecological momentary assessment in audiology research. *J. Am. Acad. Audiol.* **2015**, *26*, 872–884. [CrossRef]
31. Xu, D.; Yapanel, U.; Gray, S. Reliability of the LENATM Language Environment Analysis System in Young Children's Natural Home Environment. 2009. Available online: https://www.lena.org/wp-content/uploads/2016/07/LTR-05-2_Reliability.pdf (accessed on 30 June 2016).

32. Schvartz-Leyzac, K.C.; Conrad, C.A.; Zwolan, T.A. Datalogging Statistics and Speech Recognition during the First Year of Use in Adult Cochlear Implant Recipients. *Otol. Neurotol.* **2019**, *40*, E686–E693. [CrossRef]
33. Hey, M.; Böhnke, B.; Mewes, A.; Munder, P.; Mauger, S.J.; Hocke, T. Speech comprehension across multiple CI processor generations: Scene dependent signal processing. *Laryngoscope Investig. Otolaryngol.* **2021**, *6*, 807–815. [CrossRef]
34. Dziemba, O.C.; Merz, S.; Hocke, T. Evaluative audiometry after cochlear implant provision. *HNO* **2023**, *72*, 56–62. [CrossRef]
35. Mauger, S.J.; Warren, C.D.; Knight, M.R.; Goorevich, M.; Nel, E. Clinical evaluation of the Nucleus 6 cochlear implant system: Performance improvements with SmartSound iQ. *Int. J. Audiol.* **2014**, *53*, 564–576. [CrossRef] [PubMed]
36. Rader, T.; Doms, P.; Adel, Y.; Weissgerber, T.; Strieth, S.; Baumann, U. A method for determining precise electrical hearing thresholds in cochlear implant users. *Int. J. Audiol.* **2018**, *57*, 502–509. [CrossRef]
37. Wagener, K.; Kühnel, V.; and Kollmeier, B. Entwicklung und Evaluation eines Satztests in deutscher Sprache I–III: Design, Optimierung und Evaluation des Oldenburger Satztests. *Z. Für Audiol. /Audiol. Acoust.* **1999**, *38*, 4–15.
38. Kollmeier, B.; Warzybok, A.; Hochmuth, S.; Zokoll, M.A.; Uslar, V.; Brand, T.; Wagener, K.C. The multilingual matrix test: Principles, applications, and comparison across languages: A review. *Int. J. Audiol.* **2015**, *54*, 3–16. [CrossRef]
39. Meister, H. Speech comprehension and cognitive performance in acoustically difficult situations. *HNO* **2019**, *68*, 171–176. [CrossRef]
40. Rahne, T.; Wagner, T.M.; Kopsch, A.C.; Plontke, S.K.; Wagner, L. Influence of Age on Speech Recognition in Noise and Hearing Effort in Listeners with Age-Related Hearing Loss. *J. Clin. Med.* **2023**, *12*, 6133. [CrossRef] [PubMed]
41. Keidser, G.; Naylor, G.; Brungart, D.S.; Caduff, A.; Campos, J.; Carlile, S.; Carpenter, M.G.; Grimm, G.; Hohmann, V.; Holube, I.; et al. The Quest for Ecological Validity in Hearing Science: What It Is, Why It Matters, and How to Advance It. *Ear Hear.* **2020**, *41*, 5S–19S. [CrossRef] [PubMed]
42. Holube, I.; von Gablenz, P.; Bitzer, J. Ecological Momentary Assessment in Hearing Research: Current State, Challenges, and Future Directions. *Ear Hear.* **2020**, *41*, 79S–90S. [CrossRef]
43. Volleth, N.; Hast, A.; Lehmann, E.K.; Hoppe, U. Subjektive Hörverbesserung durch Cochleaimplantatversorgung. *HNO* **2018**, *66*, 613–620. [CrossRef]
44. Tolisano, A.M.; Pillion, E.M.; Dirks, C.E.; Ryan, M.T.; Bernstein, J.G.W. Quality of Life Impact of Cochlear Implantation for Single-Sided Deafness: Assessing the Interrelationship of Objective and Subjective Measures. *Otol. Neurotol.* **2023**, *44*, E125–E132. [CrossRef] [PubMed]
45. Plesch, J.; Ernst, B.P.; Strieth, S.; Rader, T. A psychoacoustic application for the adjustment of electrical hearing thresholds in cochlear implant patients. *PLoS ONE* **2019**, *14*, e0223625. [CrossRef] [PubMed]
46. Weissgerber, T.; Löschner, M.; Stöver, T.; Baumann, U. Outcome Prediction of Speech Perception in Quiet and in Noise for Cochlear Implant Candidates Based on Pre-Operative Measures. *J. Clin. Med.* **2024**, *13*, 994. [CrossRef]
47. Lenarz, M.; Sönmez, H.; Joseph, G.; Büchner, A.; Lenarz, T. Long-term performance of cochlear implants in postlingually deafened adults. *Otolaryngol.-Head Neck Surg.* **2012**, *147*, 112–118. [CrossRef]
48. Krueger, B.; Joseph, G.; Rost, U.; Strau-Schier, A.; Lenarz, T.; Buechner, A. Performance Groups in Adult Cochlear Implant Users. *Otol. Neurotol.* **2008**, *29*, 509–512. [CrossRef] [PubMed]
49. *ISO 8253-2*; Acoustics—Audiometric Test Methods—Part 2: Sound Field Audiometry with Pure-Tone and Narrow-Band Test Signals. International Organization for Standardization: Geneva, Switzerland, 2010. [CrossRef]
50. Hahlbrock, K. Speech audiometry and new word-tests. *Arch. Für Ohren- Nasen- Und Kehlkopfheilkd* **1953**, *162*, 394–431. [CrossRef]
51. Brand, T.; Kollmeier, B. Efficient adaptive procedures for threshold and concurrent slope estimates for psychophysics and speech intelligibility tests. *J. Acoust. Soc. Am.* **2002**, *111*, 2801–2810. [CrossRef] [PubMed]
52. Hey, M.; Hocke, T.; Hedderich, J.; Müller-Deile, J. Investigation of a matrix sentence test in noise: Reproducibility and discrimination function in cochlear implant patients. *Int. J. Audiol.* **2014**, *53*, 895–902. [CrossRef] [PubMed]
53. Deutsche Gesellschaft für Hals-Nasen-Ohren-Heilkunde Kopf- und Hals-Chirurgie e.V. (DGHNO-KHC). *S2k-Leitlinie Cochlea-Implantat Versorgung*. 2020. Available online: https://www.awmf.org/uploads/tx_szleitlinien/017-071l_S2k_Cochlea-Implantat-Versorgung-zentral-auditorische-Implantate_2020-12.pdf (accessed on 3 May 2024).
54. Rader, T.; Fastl, H.; Baumann, U. Speech perception with combined electric-acoustic stimulation and bilateral cochlear implants in a multisource noise field. *Ear Hear.* **2013**, *34*, 324–332. [CrossRef]
55. Dreschler, W.A.; Verschuure, H.; Ludvigsen, C.; Westermann, S. ICRA Noises: Artificial Noise Signals with Speech-like Spectral and Temporal Properties for Hearing Instrument Assessment. *Int. J. Audiol.* **2001**, *40*, 148–157. [CrossRef]
56. Hey, M.; Mewes, A.; Hocke, T. Speech comprehension in noise—Considerations for ecologically valid assessment of communication skills ability with cochlear implants. *HNO* **2023**, *71*, 26–34. [CrossRef]
57. Gatehouse, S.; Noble, I. The Speech, Spatial and Qualities of Hearing Scale (SSQ). *Int. J. Audiol.* **2004**, *43*, 85–99. [CrossRef]
58. Kießling, J.; Grugel, L.; Meister, H.; Meis, M. Übertragung der Fragebögen SADL, ECHO und Übertragung der Fragebögen SADL, ECHO und SSQ ins Deutsche und deren Evaluation. *ZfA* **2011**, *49*, 6–16.
59. Singh, G.; Kathleen Pichora-Fuller, M. Older adults' performance on the speech, spatial, and qualities of hearing scale (SSQ): Test-retest reliability and a comparison of interview and self-administration methods. *Int. J. Audiol.* **2010**, *49*, 733–740. [CrossRef] [PubMed]
60. Schulte, M.; Meis, M.; Wagener, K. Der Höranstrengungs-Fragebogen. 18. *Jahrestag. Der Dtsch. Ges. Für Audiol.* **2015**, *4*, 7.3.

61. Klopp, E. Explorative Faktorenanalyse. 2010. Available online: https://psycharchives.org/en/item/8bd2d5e7-0941-4198-ab23-e94e19e47223 (accessed on 3 May 2024).
62. Winkler, A.; Holube, I. Test-Retest-Reliabilität des Freiburger Einsilbertests. *HNO* **2016**, *64*, 564–571. [CrossRef] [PubMed]
63. Browning, L.M.; Nie, Y.; Rout, A.; Heiner, M. Audiologists' preferences in programming cochlear implants: A preliminary report. *Cochlear Implant. Int.* **2020**, *21*, 179–191. [CrossRef] [PubMed]
64. Busby, P.A.; Arora, K. Effects of threshold adjustment on speech perception in nucleus cochlear implant recipients. *Ear Hear.* **2016**, *37*, 303–311. [CrossRef]
65. De Graaff, F.; Lissenberg-Witte, B.I.; Kaandorp, M.W.; Merkus, P.; Goverts, S.T.; Kramer, S.E.; Smits, C. Relationship between Speech Recognition in Quiet and Noise and Fitting Parameters, Impedances and ECAP Thresholds in Adult Cochlear Implant Users. *Ear Hear.* **2020**, *41*, 935–947. [CrossRef]
66. Hinderink, J.B.; Krabbe, P.F.M.; Van Den Broek, P. Development and application of a health-related quality-of-life instrument for adults with cochlear implants: The Nijmegen Cochlear Implant Questionnaire. *Otolaryngol.-Head Neck Surg.* **2000**, *123*, 756–765. [CrossRef] [PubMed]
67. McRackan, T.R.; Bauschard, M.; Hatch, J.L.; Franko-Tobin, E.; Droghini, H.R.; Nguyen, S.A.; Dubno, J.R. Meta-analysis of quality-of-life improvement after cochlear implantation and associations with speech recognition abilities. *Laryngoscope* **2018**, *128*, 982–990. [CrossRef] [PubMed]
68. Capretta, N.R.; Moberly, A.C. Does quality of life depend on speech recognition performance for adult cochlear implant users? *Laryngoscope* **2016**, *126*, 699–706. [CrossRef] [PubMed]
69. Ovari, A.; Hühnlein, L.; Nguyen-Dalinger, D.; Strüder, D.F.; Külkens, C.; Niclaus, O.; Meyer, J.E. Functional Outcomes and Quality of Life after Cochlear Implantation in Patients with Long-Term Deafness. *J. Clin. Med.* **2022**, *11*, 5156. [CrossRef]
70. Weissgerber, T.; Rader, T.; Baumann, U. Effectiveness of directional microphones in bilateral/bimodal cochlear implant users-impact of spatial and temporal noise characteristics. *Otol. Neurotol.* **2017**, *38*, e551–e557. [CrossRef]
71. Müller, A.; Hocke, T.; Mir-Salim, P. Intraoperative findings on ECAP-measurement: Normal or special case? *Int. J. Audiol.* **2015**, *54*, 257–264. [CrossRef]
72. Hoppe, U.; Hocke, T.; Hast, A.; Iro, H. Maximum preimplantation monosyllabic score as predictor of cochlear implant outcome. *HNO* **2019**, *67*, 62–68. [CrossRef]

MDPI AG
Grosspeteranlage 5
4052 Basel
Switzerland
Tel.: +41 61 683 77 34

Journal of Clinical Medicine Editorial Office
E-mail: jcm@mdpi.com
www.mdpi.com/journal/jcm

www.ingramcontent.com/pod-product-compliance
Lightning Source LLC
Chambersburg PA
CBHW062057220926
51850CB00010B/2799
* 9 7 8 3 7 2 5 8 5 7 1 3 5 *